Amanda Hamilton and Sandy Newbigging

Life-Changing Weight Loss

3 steps to get the body and life you want

PIATKUS

PIATKUS

First published in Great Britain in 2008 by Piatkus Books
Copyright © Amanda Hamilton and Sandy Newbigging 2008
The moral right of the authors has been asserted

A CIP catalogue record for this book
is available from the British Library

ISBN 978-0-7499-2837-7

Designed by Two Associates
Printed and bound in Italy by L.E.G.O. SpA

Piatkus Books
An imprint of
Little, Brown Book Group
100 Victoria Embankment
London EC4Y 0DY

An Hachette Livre UK Company
www.hachettelivre.co.uk

www.piatkus.co.uk

While the authors have made every effort to ensure the information in this book is
accurate, it is advisory only and should not be taken as medical advice. Neither the
authors nor the publishers accept any responsibility for legal or medical liability or
other consequences which may arise directly or indirectly as a consequence of the use
or misuse of the information contained in this book.

Dedication

To everyone who has ever been trapped in the web of weight loss. May this book help in some way to set you free. **Amanda**

You are perfect, complete and beyond-words beautiful, exactly as you are now. It is my hope this book will help you realise this universal and timeless truth. **Sandy**

Acknowledgements

I would like to thank the supportive team at Little, Brown for bringing together the two aspects of the book so smoothly. From my support network, the biggest thanks is to Karen Devine for her help and humour when the deadlines got tough, but most of all for her enduring friendship. As ever, thanks to my beautiful daughter. The inspiration for this book lies in the hope that our children will be wiser than we are with their bodies and minds. And finally to Crawfurd, for tending to the fire that binds. **Amanda**

Thanks to my parents John and Sandra and brother Max for their continued support and encouragement. Thanks to all my amazing friends – I feel humbled by your ability to always see the best in me. Special thanks to Bryce Redford, Lindsey Best and Mahadeva Ishaya for your wisdom, unconditional love and, perhaps most importantly, playfulness! **Sandy**

We would like to thank Gill Bailey and Jillian Stewart at Piatkus for all of their fantastic advice and support, and our copy editor Lisa Hughes for her excellent work in editing. We would also like to thank our photographer Adam Lawrence and our designer James Empringham. **Sandy and Amanda**

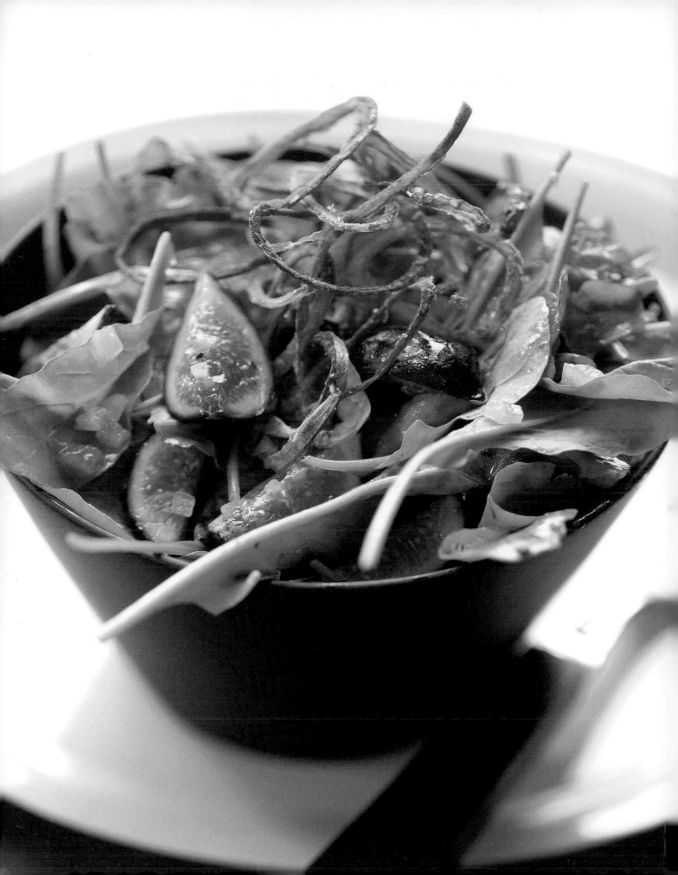

contents

Introduction

Finally, a weight loss book that combines the best of body and mind advice that can deliver remarkable, permanent results – fast! Been on and off the diet wagon? Do you break your regime under stress? Can't lose the weight you want to or do you always put it back on? It's hardly surprising when so many conventional diets tackle just one aspect of weight loss, such as restricting calories, and ignore all the other factors that affect our ability to achieve and sustain a healthy weight.

This book is different – it shows you how to overcome the hidden causes, both physical and emotional, that prevent you from getting the body you want. But the benefits don't stop there. As you embark on making positive changes to your body and your mind, it is impossible not to improve the quality and enjoyment of the rest of your life, too.

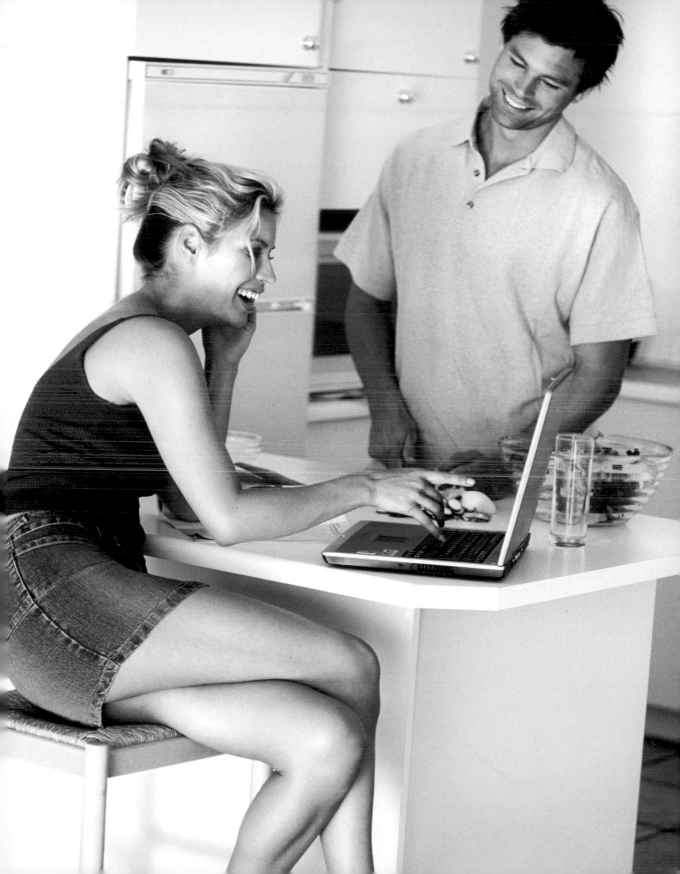

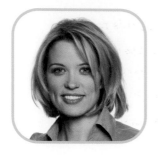

Welcome from Amanda

In my career as a nutritionist I've come up against one problem that causes more anxiety, distress and heartache than any other. That problem is weight gain and what to do about it. I run weight-loss retreats all over the world, where I teach people what you will be able to learn by reading this book – the only thing you have to do is implement my advice! My other career as a TV presenter means that I am under a lot of pressure to look good, but luckily I have learned the techniques of staying slim without having to put in too much effort. After all, who wants a life of measuring every morsel and counting every calorie – not me and, I hazard a guess, not you either!

In my experience, the 'diet industry', with all its fads, quick fixes and calorie counting, is part of the problem, not the solution. That's why this book had to be about *life-changing* weight loss – not just lose ten pounds in ten days and then put it all back on, plus more... Does that sound familiar? Are you tired of that old routine? Well, read on.

The new way to lose weight

Chances are you've been on a diet before, right? But if you're reading this it clearly didn't give you what you needed. Most diets leave the body depleted and ready to store fat again – quickly! Being able to forget about the detail of food and instead stick to the nutrient – that's right, nutrient – principle is one of the most liberating experiences of your life.

Calorie counting is hurtfully deceptive. Calories can be empty and toxic, making you crave more food, and preventing your body from burning fat and getting rid of fattening chemicals. It's like saying sprinkle this miracle fertiliser on your lawn, but take away the soil in which the grass grows. Your body is your earth. Without the right food your body can't do its work. By first helping you to reveal the hidden reasons behind your weight gain, the life-changing weight loss plan then helps you harness the power of your body and mind to lose weight.

I have seen how clients' lives are transformed when they uncover a truth about their body, how it works and why they have struggled with their weight. It's a turning point for them. It's like finding out that you've been putting diesel in a petrol engine and expecting your car to perform perfectly. Well, think about your stubborn weight gain as your body's behavioural problem! You need to understand why it is refusing to let the weight go, why the strategies you're using aren't working and how to put together a long-term system that really works. But it does mean putting in a bit of time at the beginning (not much though, as we've done most of the work for you...) to develop a proper understanding of why you are the way you are now.

The life-changing weight loss plan is designed to boost nutrition on every level, so that the body is able to manage weight effectively. Did you know that your liver is your major fat-burning organ? If it's too clogged up with toxins from man-made chemicals then it can't function optimally. Are you aware that digestion is also vital for weight management? You're not what you eat, you're what you absorb. The better your body digests and eliminates, the better 'tuned in' you are to what your body needs. Time after time I've seen how clients have not only lost (and kept off) stubborn pounds or stones, but also how their general health improves as these vital systems in the body are boosted.

How life-changing weight loss will boost your body

This eating plan is jam-packed full of nutrient-rich foods that provide life-promoting vitamins, minerals and essential fats – and all the foods are easy to get hold of and prepare. This is not about depriving you of good tasting food, it's about increasing your enjoyment of natural flavours and letting your body work better than it has in years. Natural wholefoods, such as good quality proteins, wholegrains, seeds, nuts, fruits and vegetables give the body proper nutrition, which keeps you mentally, emotionally and physically balanced. Small amounts of protein taken with each meal slow down the release of sugar in the body and keep you feeling full for longer. Essential fats slow down the transit of foods and also help the body absorb nutrients better. They're also needed by the liver in its job of metabolising fat – you need to eat good fat to burn bad fat!

So, ditch the calorie counting and instead turn to nutrient maxing! In essence, what this means is making sure that the majority of what you consume is of the highest nutritional quality, but at the same time you need to take out the 'nutrient robbers' – the pre-packed, processed, chemically altered foods that all add to your body's toxic load. The more toxins the body takes in, the more difficult it is for it to manage weight effectively.

The longer term results of eating nutrient-rich food are more energy and vitality, better skin, better concentration and mood, and effortless weight control. After all, human beings are not meant to be overweight – it's merely a symptom of a toxic lifestyle, whether indirectly through a hidden problem or directly through what you eat and drink. Eventually, you'll find that you naturally and effortlessly 'tune' into your body's needs and listen to the foods your body requires for health and vitality, instead of feeding the craving for addictive substances.

My approach to weight loss has evolved over the years, as I've taken my medical studies and nutritional research and combined them with a hefty dose of 'real life'. These days I don't tell my own clients to diet. Instead, I use this plan to help them follow the tune their body and mind dances to. That's why *Life-Changing Weight Loss* can make the difference for you. Find your rhythm again, understand how your body works and begin emerging as your true, slim self.

Amanda

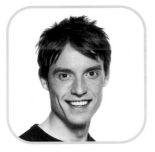

Welcome from Sandy

You may have wanted to lose weight for some time now. You may have tried different diets and been disappointed with the long-term results. I appreciate that this can be disheartening and cause you to question your ability to have the body you want. However, irrespective of what's happened in the past, you need to leave the past where it belongs – in the past!

I can say this because I'm a therapist or, to be more accurate, a mind detox therapist. I have clinics in Edinburgh and London, and I run popular retreats, in the UK and overseas, that take a mind-and-body approach to healing and happiness. I also do a certain amount of TV work and have appeared on three series of UKTV's *Spa of Embarrassing Illnesses*. These programmes, which have aired in over 30 countries around the world, have shown how I help people to 'change their mind' in order to transform their body and their life, so please believe me when I say that assuming your past inevitably equals your future, or that you can't change your body, is simply not true. The fact is you are constantly changing, physically, mentally and emotionally.

Let this moment be a new beginning

When it comes to your body, millions of remarkable changes are happening 24 hours a day, seven days a week. Every second ten million of your cells die and are immediately replaced by ten million new ones. Every five days you create a new stomach lining, every month you create a new skin, every six weeks you generate a new liver and during every three months you even 'grow' a new skeleton! But the changes don't stop there. Radioactive isotope studies have found that we replace almost all (98%) of the atoms of our body every year.

On top of these miraculous physical changes, every day you have around 100,000 thoughts, a whole range of emotions and make countless choices that all add up to making the 'you' that you see in the mirror. So it isn't a matter of *if* you can change, because you're constantly changing. Every second offers the gift of a new beginning; a new opportunity to take charge of your physical and emotional destiny, and use your mind to help you lose weight.

Changing your mind changes your body

A commonly held misconception in the western world is that the mind and body are separate entities – that there are physical problems and there are emotional problems. However, the mind and body are very much one entity. When you change your mind, your body responds accordingly, because the mind and body are connected and in constant communication with each other. Within the following pages I will explain the mind–body connection in easy-to-understand terms, and share proven and powerful exercises to help you harness its power in order to lose weight.

My approach has always been to work with my clients to help them get to the root causes of their problems, instead of dealing solely with the surface-level symptoms. Weight loss is no different. I have found repeatedly that excess weight is never *the* problem, but rather a symptom of one or more physical and/or emotional problems.

Human bodies are programmed for survival. Your body has gained weight in an attempt to adapt to, and survive, the physical and emotional conditions it's been subjected to throughout your life. For you to successfully lose weight you need to become aware of the reasons *why* your body has felt the need to adapt by gaining weight, and then make a few changes to the physical and emotional conditions in which your body exists. Doing so will cause your body to adapt again, but this time by losing weight.

My approach comes with a caveat though, which is to keep an open mind. Remember, if you always do what you've always done, you will always get what you've always got! Some of my methods may be new to you and at first glance you could find yourself questioning how certain mental blocks or emotional issues could lead to weight gain. Nevertheless, I ask you to suspend judgement, trust the process and let the results speak for themselves – the proof is in the pudding, as they say!

About this book

Weight gain doesn't just impact on your appearance, it can be a serious health risk. Obesity levels, which are already dangerously high, are rising at an alarming rate and the associated health problems, such as heart disease, diabetes, cancer and stroke, top the league tables of deadly diseases. There has never been a more important time to be proactive about getting the body you want.

Healthy body + healthy mind = long-term weight loss

A healthy body plus a healthy mind is the ideal formula for long-term weight loss. As a result, this book is specially designed to help you create and enjoy both. Most diets starve the body of the very nutrients it needs to become healthy. This book is different, because it provides nutritional guidelines that help your body build up reserves of the essential nutrients which it needs to help to metabolise fats and maintain vitality, and it helps you to resolve the emotional problems that could cause you to eat comfort foods in excess.

Our holistic 3-step approach

Our 3-step approach works so successfully because we take a mind-and-body approach to weight loss and help you to:

Step 1   Discover the hidden physical and emotional reasons why you weigh what you do

Step 2   Resolve the reasons for your excess weight

Step 3   Enjoy life as you naturally and quickly lose weight

By approaching weight loss with our holistic three-step plan, you will benefit from greater overall physical, mental, emotional and spiritual health and well-being. We have found that sustained weight loss is the natural by-product of a person who has become happier in their own skin, prioritised their health and is enjoying the life they want. This is why we call our plan *life-changing* weight loss – we've found people rarely lose weight without changing their life for the better.

Benefits beyond weight loss

It is not just in the prevention of serious health problems that your body will feel the benefit of this life-changing weight loss programme. Healthy weight loss helps digestive complaints such as bloating become a thing of the past. Your skin will glow and your energy will increase, not to mention the mental freedom that you'll experience when the shackles of the depressing diet cycle are finally shaken off. Are you ready to begin?

The life-changing laws

You can take charge of your physical and emotional destiny and this book can show you how. In order to get the greatest benefit from what we suggest it is vital you follow these life-changing laws:

Be here now

Never postpone health and happiness to some point in the future, because now is the ONLY time you can enjoy either. Decisions to change your body or your life can only happen 'in the now', because this moment, right here, right now, is the only time you can do anything. Your life consists of nothing more than the continuous present you're in. When you're living in the moment you're free from past problems and future worries, and able to make decisions and take actions consistent with what you want – now. Don't wait until some time in the future to decide and act. Take charge of your health and happiness now… and now… and now!

Resolve the root-cause reason

You can have the body and life you want by resolving the root-cause reasons for your current body and life problems. We specialise in helping people to find what we call the root-cause reasons for their physical health conditions and problematic life circumstances. Root-cause reasons tend to exist and operate in the realms of your mind that you're not consciously aware of. This can make them very difficult to find and fix – unless you know how. Our approach finds the root-cause reasons and then shows you how to resolve them. We have repeatedly found that if you discover *why* you have a weight problem, then it is inevitable that you will succeed in shifting that excess weight for good. Imagine that!

Be committed to what you want

What's your IQ level? By that, we mean your 'I quit' level? What is it going to take for you to give up? Making a commitment has the power to turn the possibility of you getting the body you want into an inevitability.

Commitment requires you to do the things you said you would, long after the positive emotions you had when you said you would do them have left you. A genuine commitment allows for no get-out clause or any ifs, buts or maybes – just the total acceptance that you will take persistent action until you get what you want. It also makes getting your ideal body and life inevitable, because instead of focusing on whether you do it, you can focus your energy and attention on why you want it, how you're going to do it and all the ways you can enjoy the process.

Make a commitment to yourself now by writing out and signing a statement similar to this:

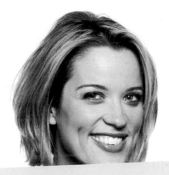

Life-changing weight loss commitment

I hereby commit to take charge of my body by being my ideal weight. I will persist until I succeed, and have lots of fun doing it!

Signed:..

Date:...............................

Motivation for long-term weight loss

You're motivated enough to lose weight to buy this book, but are you motivated for life-changing weight loss? By this we mean are you only interested in a quick fix or do you genuinely want to enjoy your ideal body for life?

Check your motives

Be ruthlessly honest with yourself about your motives for losing weight. Are you solely motivated to be slimmer for a short-term external event? If so, then your motivation can disappear once that event has passed. By all means use such events or goals to prompt positive change but it is important to realise that in order to achieve and maintain long-term weight loss, as opposed to just a short-term drop in weight, you need to back up those goals with a commitment to achieving better health and happiness for yourself. If you are motivated by the following short-term goals, think about how you can use that drive to achieve long-term success:

- **To keep up appearances** Having a desire to look healthy is great, but being driven to lose weight *only* to look better to others can mean your motivation disappears the moment you look in the mirror and like what you see. If you also recognise how much better you *feel* once you've lost weight it will help you realise how important health is.
- **To slim for a special event** Wanting to lose weight for a special event, such as a wedding or a holiday, is common and can cause you to be highly motivated for a short period of time, but be careful not to slip back to your old 'unhealthy' ways once the date has passed. Why not think of the whole of your life as the 'special event' you want to be your best for – after all it's the only life you've got!
- **To feel happy** Advertising, media and marketing campaigns all play their part in promoting the myth that having a 'beautiful body' will mean you'll automatically be happier. It's simply not the case.

Happiness is a state of being that you can access at any moment, irrespective of your physical shape or weight.

- **To meet that special someone** Improving your looks in order to attract a mate is natural. However, again, it can lead to only short-term motivation that disappears when you meet that special someone.
- **To rescue a failing relationship** Losing weight to fix a problematic relationship can result in resentment building up towards the other person. It can also lead to the unhealthy behaviours returning if you don't get the responses and results you want.
- **To become loveable** Genuine self-love is unconditional, so if you lose weight to love yourself then you will probably find you don't love the slimmer you either. Every human being is divine and it is your birthright to know you are loveable, exactly as you are now.

None of these externally focused motives are necessarily bad or wrong, we are simply recommending you also aim to motivate yourself by some internally focused reasons, too; for instance, because you want to take care of your body, because your body deserves to be treated with love and respect or because you want to be a healthy and active parent. When you love and value yourself, you naturally gravitate towards being, doing and having what is best for your body and your life (see pages 71–73 for more on how to love yourself), and we have found that when a person loves and respects their body, then starting and sticking to a life-changing programme like ours becomes both natural and effortless.

On a piece of paper or in a notebook, write down a list of the top three reasons why you want to lose weight. Having a mix of both short- and long-term, and externally and internally focused motivators, increases the likelihood of sustaining the amazing benefits you could reap from this book.

Using this book

Life-Changing Weight Loss is divided into three steps.

In **Step 1** you discover why you weigh what you do by exploring the physical and emotional causes of your current shape and weight.

In **Step 2** you move on to resolve them. This is accomplished by first exploring the physical factors involved in long-term weight loss and then progressing to complete proven and powerful 'mind exercises' that can help you to resolve the main emotional causes of weight gain. In Step 2 there is also a seven-day, kick-start life-changing weight loss plan to get you off to the best possible start.

Finally, **Step 3** looks at some of the issues you may face continuing the plan and shares some top tips for maintaining it, so that you can enjoy the body you want for life.

Don't skip straight to the eating plan. Many people do this with diet books but this isn't your average diet book and you have some work to do in Step 1 before you can begin to resolve your problems. When you reach Step 2 you can either work through the exercises in the order they appear or you can use the seven-day kick-start plan, which directs you to different mind exercises each day, as your guide.

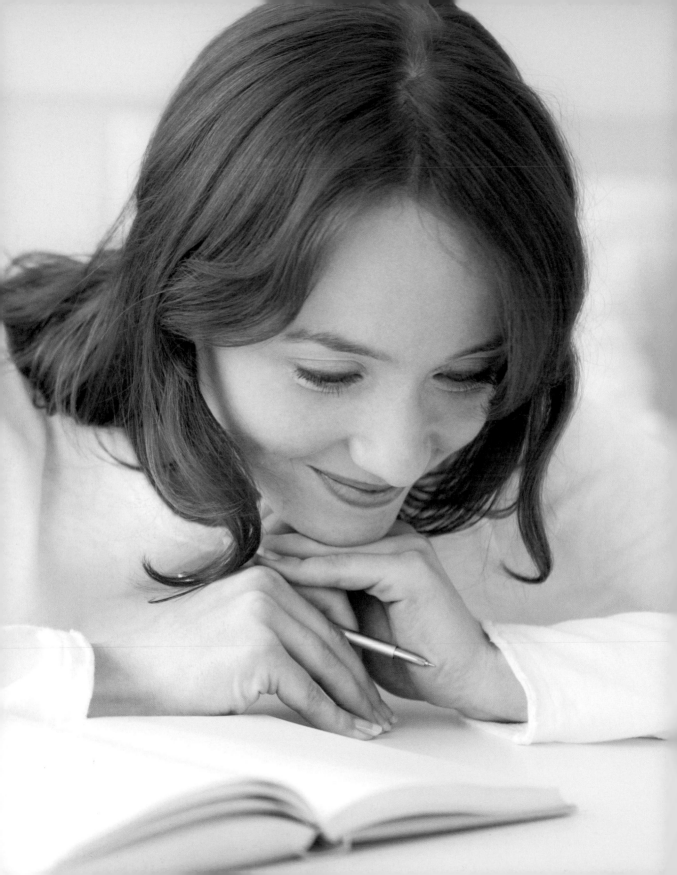

Step 1: Discover
why you weigh what you do

The chances are, if you've been unsuccessful at permanently losing weight in the past, it's because you haven't yet resolved the hidden reasons behind *why* your body gained weight in the first place. Step 1 is all about helping you to discover the physical and emotional causes of your weight gain, so you can move on to resolve them – and lose the excess weight, too – once and for all.

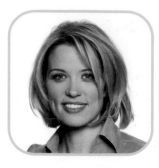

For the body: Do some groundwork

If you're like most people you'll be tempted to rush straight to the eating plan in Step 2, but I highly recommend you use this book in the order in which it is set out and first discover and resolve the main physical and emotional reasons for your current body shape and weight. Doing this will give you with the best possible chance to keep the excess weight off, for life!

To create the right conditions to lose weight, forever, you need to get to know your body type. Maybe you've never considered yourself a type – after all, it does sound rather like dating! However, understanding which of the three body types you are gives you a realistic body shape to aim for and means you can choose the right weight loss strategies; the ones that are most likely to work for you and your body type.

What body type are you?

If you look at the people around you'll start to see that there are different types of body. Most medical systems, both ancient and modern, use body typing as a way to help to classify individual predispositions to weight gain, certain illnesses and even personality traits. To help identify my clients' body types, I draw on the body typing systems of Ayurveda, the 'science of life' from India, as well as the Western medical ectomorph (naturally slender), mesomorph (medium build, athletic) and endomorph (larger build, curvy or heavier) classifications.

It is important to recognise that *any* of the body types can gain weight, but that each gain – and lose – weight in slightly different ways. If you're interested in life-changing weight loss you need to understand what your natural, healthy body type is – and you need to aim for a return to your own body type, not someone else's!

Meet the Kate Moss/Mick Jagger type. If this is your natural body state then you are slim, and often have long legs and arms. You're likely to have highly visible veins on your arms and hands – not just on the top of your hands, where everyone can see their veins, but on the palms. You are probably also prone to wind, constipation, and dry skin and hair. In mental and emotional terms, this body type is generally creative and changeable. Any weight gain you experience is likely to be around your middle, but you tend to be able to lose weight easily. However, you need to introduce routine and structure to support your new way of life, as practicalities can often be left to the last minute. Sandy is this body type.

Next, meet the Steffi Graff/Andre Agassi type. If this is your natural body state then you are of medium height and build, with good muscle tone – the classic athlete. Given your natural physicality, you were probably quite competitive and sporty in your youth. On the mental and emotional side, this body type is often ambitious and driven, sometimes to the detriment of their health, and can be irritable when out of balance. Unless there is an underlying medical issue, you tend to gain weight gradually and it will be distributed evenly over your body. Your weight loss is usually steady and is best supported by a focused exercise programme, but you shouldn't get too hung up on what it says on the scales, since this body type has a propensity to build muscle and muscle is about 18 per cent denser and heavier than fat. Amanda is this body type.

Finally, meet the Marilyn Monroe/Russell Crowe type. If this is your natural body state then you are of heavier build and more prone to weight gain. Women are likely to have plenty of natural curves – the classic pear shape – and men are likely to be stockier, no matter what their height. Both men and women of this type can be prone to sluggishness, although when active or working out their endurance is very good. Mentally and emotionally this type is the classic follower and

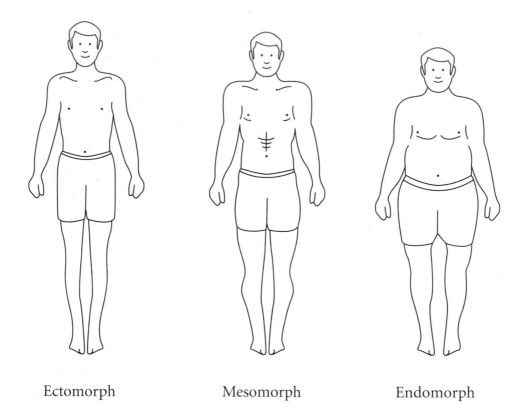

Ectomorph   Mesomorph   Endomorph

friend, loyal and more cautious than the other two. If this is your body type you'll need to take consistent care in order to prevent significant weight gain, although remember that you'll always be naturally more rounded, so celebrate those curves! If you are this body type then try to introduce regular exercise and keep to the menu planner as much as possible for optimum, healthy weight loss.

How much should you weigh?

As you've probably gathered, I believe that your body type can determine what is a healthy weight range for you, so the best policy is probably to note down changes – hopefully reductions – in your trouser or dress measurements and enjoy the increased energy that results from the life-changing weight loss plan.

For women, a waist measurement of 80 to 88cm (31.5 to 34.6in) is high and over 88cm is very high. For men, a waist measurement of 94 to 102cm (37 to 40in) is high and above that very high. A large waist measurement indicates the presence of unhealthy internal fat.

However, many of you will want to go a step further and calculate your body mass index or BMI. This is a measure of how much fat you're carrying using a calculation that takes into account your weight and height. Bear in mind that any variation within the 'healthy' category is fine. For example, a BMI of 19 is no better than 23 for a woman who's 1.6m (5ft 3in) tall, as the range takes different body types into account.

How to calculate your BMI

Weigh yourself first thing in the morning on an empty stomach or at least a couple of hours after any food. Wear minimal clothing and make sure your shoes are off. Weight fluctuates from day to day and in women it varies throughout the hormonal cycle, so these factors should be taken into account.

To calculate your BMI take your height in metres and square it (multiply the figure by itself). Measure your weight in kilograms and divide your weight by your height squared. For example, if you're 1.6m (5ft 3in) tall and weigh 65kg (10 stone), the calculation would be:

1.6 x 1.6 = 2.56
65 ÷ 2.56 = 25.39

In this example, the person has a BMI of 25.39, so she's overweight, but not by much. A BMI of 18.5 to 25 is normal, 25 to 30 is overweight, 30 to 40 is obese and over 40 is severely obese. A BMI of less than 18.5 is officially classed as underweight.

Diets don't work

The very fact that you're reading this book means you haven't yet found a 'diet' that helps you lose weight and keep it off. That's because the truth is that diets don't work in the long term.

Many 'fad' diets aren't nutritionally balanced, so they starve the body of the vital nutrients that your body needs. Your body struggles to function without those nutrients and you may experience side-effects such as bloating, fatigue and often anxiety. On a basic level, these problems can make it very hard for you to stick to the diet.

Likewise, 'crash' diets tend to drastically restrict your body's intake of calories. Again, your body isn't getting the nutrients it needs and the result can be irritability, depression and even lowered brain function, all of which inevitably affect your motivation to continue with the diet.

In both cases, when you come off the diet, you quickly return to your previous weight and may end up gaining even more weight. This is because, lacking the nutrients it needs, your brain thinks there has been a famine and has instructed your body to store fat.

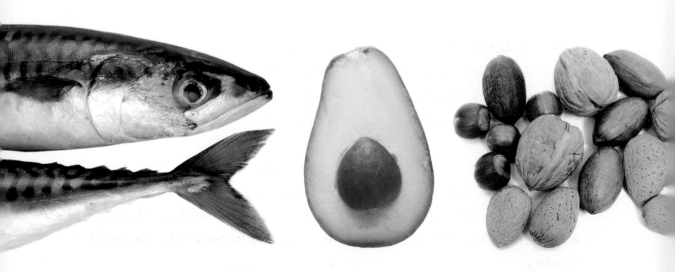

The good and bad fat guide

Fat	Type	Provides	Ideal intake
Flaxseed oil	polyunsaturated	omega-3	high
Sunflower oil	polyunsaturated	omega-6	moderate
Corn oil	polyunsaturated	omega-6	moderate
Olive oil	monounsaturated	omega-9	moderate
Soybean oil	polyunsaturated	omega-6	moderate
Lard	saturated	–	zero
Palm oil	saturated	–	zero
Coconut oil	saturated	–	moderate
Butterfat (the fat in diary products)	saturated	–	zero
Hydrogenated fat (found in processed foods)	saturated	–	zero

The need for nutrients

We need nutrients, including certain kinds of fats, to survive. The natural fats found in avocados, seeds, nuts, coconuts, oily fish etc are fats that the body recognises – particularly the omega-3, but also the omega-6 and omega-9, essential fats.

   The body uses these natural fats to generate energy, stimulate immune function and to help us 'burn' brown (adipose) fat in the body. Restricting nutrients slows down the metabolism. Without essential nutrients the glands and organs of the body, which are the main players in weight loss, are depleted of energy.

When we starve the body of nutrients, we also are more likely to experience cravings. For instance, when we are zinc-, chromium-, magnesium- and manganese-deficient we are more likely to crave sugar. This means we want foods that will raise our blood sugar levels quickly. The trouble is, the sugar in those foods tends to be stored away by our bodies equally quickly and our blood sugar levels fall sharply again, which triggers a craving for more 'false energy' from stimulants. This doesn't promote healthiness or weight loss.

Chemical calories

You may ask how on earth chemicals can cause us to gain weight. After all, they're calorie-free, aren't they? Let me explain how the process works. Honestly, once you grasp this it will change the way you eat forever!

It is an undisputed fact that there has been and continues to be a huge increase in the levels of chemicals present in our environment. At the current time it is estimated that 2,000 new industrial chemical substances make their way into our bodies each year, through the food we eat, the water we drink and the air we breathe.

These toxic chemicals include, but are not limited to:

1. Food additives, flavourings and colourings
2. Household and personal cleaning chemicals, which are both inhaled and absorbed via the skin
3. Agricultural chemicals, such as pesticides, fungicides and herbicides
4. Heavy metals, which occur naturally, but are poisonous
5. Oestrogens, which enter the environment due to human usage of the contraceptive pill and HRT
6. Xeno-oestrogens, which are chemicals that mimic oestrogen, such as dioxins.

We come into contact with thousands of new chemicals every year. These new chemicals are tested for their individual safety in the confines of a lab, but when they combine in our bodies no one really knows what the long-term effects will be.

Toxic levels of chemicals can certainly build up in our bodies, but because the human body communicates via nerve impulses and hormones, even lower levels of chemicals can interfere with our chemistry. Weight loss is controlled by the brain, because it instructs the body when to store fat and when to use fat as an energy source. Therefore, chemicals that disrupt the delicate hormonal balance of our bodies – some can even mimic our hormones – and interfere with the natural regulation of our weight will make us more susceptible to weight gain.

Many of these chemicals remain in the environment and in our food chain for an indefinite period of time. We are all touched by them or, to be more specific, our liver is touched by them.

The liver and weight gain

The liver is your main organ of detoxification and it breaks down fat in the body. If it's congested with man-made chemicals or isn't getting certain nutrients from the food you eat, the liver isn't able to work effectively. The liver needs a magic substance called bile, that yellowish-green substance, to dissolve and absorb fats. If this bile lacks nutrients or if the bile ducts themselves become blocked, then you have what is called a 'sluggish' or 'fatty' liver. A toxic or overloaded liver cannot metabolise or break down fats correctly, so it can actually cause weight gain.

Unhealthy eating means that not only are you not getting enough of the vitamins, minerals and essential fats that your body needs to work well, but also that the toxins in the food you eat can drain your body of essential nutrients – it's a vicious toxic cycle.

Social stimulants

Social stimulants are those factors or foods that are so common in our everyday lives that we fail to see them as a problem. They often fall under the weight loss radar, but without an awareness of the impact they have on weight gain you're missing a big trick. Sugar, salt, caffeine, alcohol and cigarettes are the main culprits that you need to look at for life-changing weight loss.

Sugar

Far from being a friend for work, rest and play, for anyone who wants to lose weight sugar is one of the most toxic substances around. Put simply, if you want to lose weight for life you *have* to give up sugar; it is a special occasion food only.

You may have heard of blood sugar before, perhaps in reference to diabetes or the glycemic index (GI), and keeping your blood sugar steady is vital for weight loss. However, controlling blood sugar is easy when you understand the differing effect simple and complex carbohydrates have on the body once you've consumed them. In essence, simple carbohydrates promote weight gain, whereas complex carbohydrates help you maintain or even lose weight.

Sugar – white or brown – is a simple carbohydrate. Examples of other simple carbohydrates include fruit juice, white bread, biscuits, cakes, honey, molasses and maple syrup. Simple carbohydrates, which are also known as refined sugars, are often hidden within 'diet' or 'low fat' products, so you must get label-savvy in order to detect them. These simple carbohydrates are broken down and digested very quickly, and contain very few essential vitamins and minerals.

Examples of complex carbohydrates include vegetables, wholemeal breads, pulses, brown rice and wholemeal pasta. Complex carbohydrates take longer to digest and are packed with fibre, vitamins and minerals – all of which are helpful for life-changing weight loss.

Why is it so important to choose one type of carbohydrate over

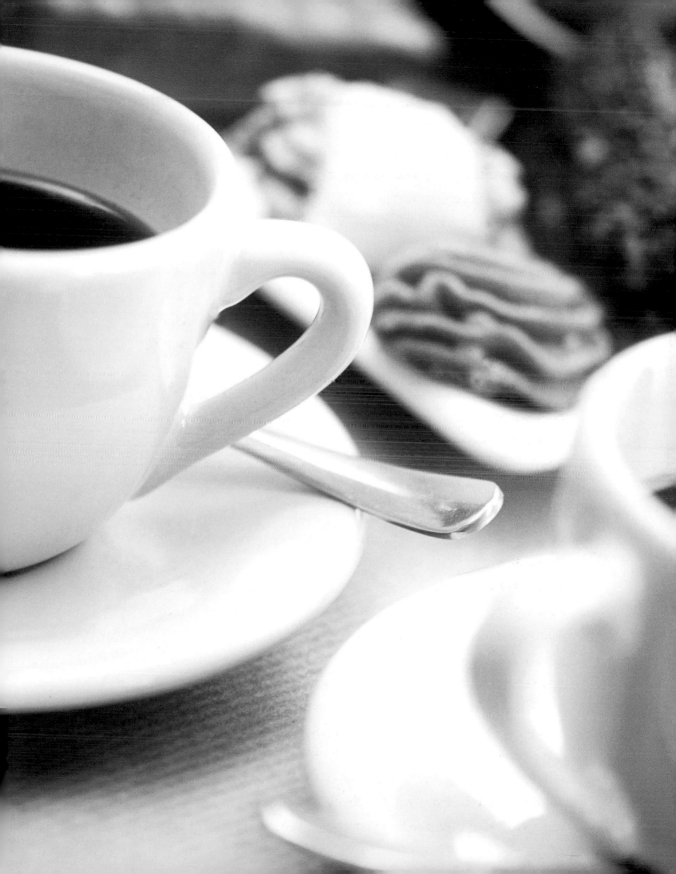

another? When you eat a simple carbohydrate, an alarm is triggered that tells your body there is sugar in your blood. Your body responds to this sudden rush of sugar by releasing a hormone called insulin, which brings down your blood sugar levels by putting a form of sugar called glucose into either your cells, where it is burnt as energy, or into your liver or muscles for storage. So far, so straightforward, right? The trouble is, when you eat a lot of sugar regularly, this insulin response becomes overloaded, resulting in the sugar being more readily stored as fat. This is how eating simple carbohydrates rather than complex carbohydrates can lead to weight gain.

Unfortunately the sugar story doesn't end there. Every time a simple carbohydrate triggers the release of insulin in your body, your cells have to react. However, if the presence of sugar in your blood becomes the norm, rather than an infrequent and special occurrence, over time your cells tire of this constant demand and become less sensitive to the insulin. This means glucose is not put into the cells, where it can be used up and burnt, so more of the sugary food you eat is stored as fat. To add insult to injury, the final blow to weight loss is that insulin is also known to hinder the stored fat from being burnt as an energy source. In other words, not only does sugar make you fatter, it will keep you that way!

Salt

The organic salt or sodium found naturally in plants is not the same as the salt or sodium chloride that is used in food manufacturing or table salt. Processed salt displaces or 'washes out' other nutrients from the body's cells. These nutrients are needed for blood sugar control and water balance, so after consuming salt you are much more likely to crave substances that give you a 'quick fix' (usually more of the salty snack you were eating... one pop, just can't stop...) and you will feel thirsty. Thirst is often mistaken for hunger so, guess what, you *eat more!* Excess salt is also known to contribute towards high blood pressure.

Caffeine

We are all familiar with the 'buzz' that caffeine can give. Many products are marketed solely on the basis of this false energy kick, but that lively feeling is actually the sensation of adrenaline being pumped around the body as a result of the caffeine hit. Much like the cells in the sugar story, the adrenal glands tire of constant stimulation and when the inevitable adrenal fatigue kicks in it leads to a slow-down in the conversion of stored fats (and proteins and carbohydrates) into energy.

We experience this failure in the energy chain as a craving for more stimulants in the form of more caffeine from another cup of tea, coffee, cola drink or caffeinated beverage. The last piece of the picture with caffeine is what it usually comes with. An average coffee these days comes with a sizeable portion of milk, sugar or syrup and then there's the ubiquitous question of whether to have a muffin or pastry with it. Cut out the caffeine and cut yourself an easier path to weight loss.

Alcohol

As far as your body is concerned, alcohol is chemically similar to sugar, so drinking any form of alcohol will set off the blood sugar seesaw that promotes weight gain. And that's before you even begin to consider the calorie content of the drink itself, which is likely to be very high and devoid of any nutritional benefit – so called 'empty calories'. What's more, alcohol acts as a potent appetite booster, so more alcohol equals more food consumed!

However, excessive calories are not the sole reason behind alcohol's 'beer belly' effect. What alcohol does is to reduce the amount of fat your body burns for energy, while preventing the absorption of many of the essential nutrients needed for successful weight loss, particularly the B vitamins and vitamin C.

According to a study carried out by the *American Journal of Clinical Nutrition*, eight men were given two drinks of vodka and sugar-free lemonade, 30 minutes apart. Each drink contained just under 90 calories. Fat metabolism was measured before and after consumption of the drink. For several hours after drinking the vodka, the men's whole body lipid oxidation, which is a measure of how much fat your body is burning, dropped by a massive 73 per cent. Because your body uses more than one source of fuel, if alcohol is consumed then this alcohol 'energy' will be used instead of fat.

For men who yearn for a muscular physique, alcohol is also bad news, as it's also one of the most effective ways to slash your testosterone levels. Just a single bout of heavy drinking raises levels of the muscle-wasting hormone cortisol and increases the breakdown of testosterone for up to 24 hours – so if you want a muscular physique, ditch the alcohol!

Cigarettes

Finally, cigarettes are another stimulant that affects the blood sugar balance. They also drain the body of vital nutrients and can even build up insulin resistance. The nicotine in cigarettes can raise the body's blood sugar levels by as much as 30 per cent, and this rapid increase is inevitably followed by a rapid drop shortly afterwards, which explains the addictive nature of nicotine.

It also explains why people giving up cigarettes often gain weight, as they satisfy their blood-sugar cravings with sweet foods rather than nicotine. Instead, if you are giving up, you should use nutritional support to balance your blood sugar and eliminate the cravings themselves.

Nicotine increases the levels of stress hormones in the body, too. If your lifestyle is stressful as well, this toxic combination can lead to imbalances in your stress hormones and may exhaust the adrenal glands that make stress hormones, leading to fatigue.

Even though cigarettes may act as an appetite suppressant in the short term, giving them up will allow your body to work towards weight loss in a healthy, long-term manner.

Underlying medical problems

Over the years, underlying medical problems often disguise themselves as symptoms of a busy lifestyle and are ignored, but for a proportion of people they hold the key to weight loss. Few people make the link between how well the body works and how easy it is to lose weight (and keep it off), but if you think about it, how can a body that is under stress metabolise fat and balance weight optimally? Once a problem is recognised it can be dealt with, so please read the sections below and if you recognise any of the problems, take the self-help test to clarify it and then take steps towards positive long-term treatment.

Underactive thyroid

Most people vaguely know there can be a link between the thyroid and weight gain, but they don't really know what might be going on and what to do about it.

The thyroid is a gland in your neck, which sits above your collar bones, in front of your windpipe. It is part of what is known as the endocrine system, which means that the hormones that are produced here are excreted directly into your bloodstream.

The thyroid produces several hormones, but the two most connected to weight gain and loss are called T4 (thyroxine) and T3 (tiiodothyronine). The thyroid gland produces up to four times as much T4 as T3, but T3, which is used to produce energy and heat, is the more active hormone. The liver, which as you now know is the organ primarily responsible for metabolising fat, has the job, along with other tissues in the body, of converting the T4 to T3. When any link in this chain fails to work optimally, it can result in weight gain.

You may have heard the term 'underactive thyroid', which is when the problem becomes so serious that drugs are needed to do what the thyroid is failing to do. However, wouldn't it make so much more sense to pick up a problem *before* drugs are required to sort it out? Many people with an underactive thyroid don't have a problem that's serious enough to be picked up by conventional testing, but the problem is still there. Have a look at the following list of symptoms, all of which can be linked to an underactive thyroid. If you suffer from a number of these symptoms there is a possibility you could have a thyroid problem so follow through on the action points in Step 2 (see page 63).

• Weight gain, even on a low-calorie or low-fat diet
• Difficulty getting warm
• Lack of energy
• Depression
• Constipation
• Dry skin and hair
• Flaking, breaking nails
• Consistently low temperature
• Frequent colds with slow recovery
• Poor circulation
• Digestive problems
• Period problems
• Loss of sex drive

The thyroid appears to be very sensitive to environmental toxic exposure, particularly smoking, as cigarettes contain high levels of cadmium, which robs you of key nutrients needed by the thyroid, so that's another good reason to stub it out.

For the thyroid to work optimally, it needs nutrients such as iodine, manganese, vitamin C, methionine, magnesium, selenium, zinc, and the amino acids cysteine and L-Tyrosine. They are all found in healthy foods such as fruit, vegetables, nuts, seeds and meat, and they not only support the gland, but also produce the thyroid hormones. Other factors, such as underlying genetic factors or traumas such as whiplash or head injury, can also play a role in weakening the thyroid.

Digestive dysfunction

As we've said before, you're not what you eat, you're what you absorb. When the body isn't breaking down food well the result is an increase in the body's toxic load, which impacts on the liver, the body's main fat-metabolising organ.

Digestion is of particular significance because of the frequency at which problems occur. In the UK, an estimated one in four people suffer from irritable bowel syndrome (IBS), but digestive dysfunction can include leaky gut syndrome, haemorrhoids and constipation. Symptoms of digestive complaints can be quite variable and include abdominal pain, bloating, and sometimes bouts of diarrhoea and/or constipation. Symptoms tend to 'come and go', often with emotional undertones, but one thing is clear: if problems are ignored, they develop into more chronic, serious conditions such as colitis or diverticulitis, so if you're suffering, make sure you see a nutritionist.

The key aspect of digestion that affects weight gain is stomach acid, which is essentially hydrochloric acid, because this is needed to break down proteins. The absorption of nutrients, particularly iron and calcium, is dependent on it and many people have a lack of stomach acid as a result of overindulgence in processed foods.

Put simply, if your digestion is not functioning optimally, then nutrients are not being absorbed optimally, which leads you to feel you're lacking something. This can translate as a simple desire for more food, because the better your body absorbs the less food it will ask for!

However, there is also a link between digestive dysfunction, and allergies and intolerances, which are other known factors in weight gain. Two-thirds of IBS sufferers have been found to have hidden food intolerances. If you suffer from digestive problems the best course of action is to take a food intolerance test which you can administer easily at home (see pages 41 and 66 for more on allergies).

Adrenal fatigue

Adrenals play a vital role in blood sugar control, thyroid output and weight control. If you have had repeated stress in your life then your adrenals may need extra support through what you eat and also certain nutritional supplements. Inappropriate levels of the cortisol, which is produced in response to stress, affect our mental, emotional and physical well-being and can lead indirectly to weight problems.

Symptoms of adrenal overload include not being able to sleep or waking up in the middle of the night, fatigue in the mornings, afternoon slumps, cravings for carbs and sugars, a desire for stimulants such as coffee and chocolate, irritability, not being able to shake off colds or finish jobs, and many more.

The good news is that adrenal fatigue can almost always be relieved. However, understanding the role of adrenals and the key cause of adrenal fatigue – stress – is vital if you want to fight stubborn weight gain.

To understand how adrenal fatigue develops, it is important to understand the original, evolutionary function of the adrenal glands. The adrenals are walnut-sized glands located on top of each kidney and they are important control centres for many of the body's hormones. The outer layer of the gland, called the adrenal cortex, produces various hormones, including cortisol, dehydroepiandrosterone (DHEA), which moderates the balance of hormones in your body, oestrogen and testosterone. The centres of the glands produce adrenaline, the hormone named after them.

The basic task of your adrenal glands is to rush all your body's resources into 'fight or flight' mode by increasing production of adrenaline and other hormones. When healthy, your adrenals can instantly increase your heart rate and blood pressure, release your energy stores for immediate use, slow your digestion and other secondary functions, and sharpen your senses. With adrenal overload the problem is not the function of the adrenals, but the overuse of them.

Unlike our ancestors, we live with constant stress. Instead of occasional, acute demands followed by rest, we're constantly overworked, under-nourished, exposed to environmental toxins, worrying about others, with no let-up. Every challenge to the mind and body creates a demand on the adrenal glands and the result is that your adrenal glands are in a state of constant high alert. This creates high levels of cortisol in the body, which leads to a wide range of health problems, including an inability to shift weight.

Sustained high levels of cortisol, triggered off by stress, gradually wears your body down. When the adrenals are chronically overworked and straining to maintain high cortisol levels, they lose the capacity to produce DHEA in sufficient amounts. Inadequate levels of DHEA contribute to fatigue, bone loss, muscle mass loss, depression, aching joints, decreased sex drive and impaired immune function, as well as thyroid problems and weight gain. If you recognise the symptoms of adrenal fatigue in yourself, then make sure you follow through on the action points in Step 2 (see page 64).

Allergies

If your body is responding to an allergy or intolerance it will often retain water. You may not know you have food intolerances; indeed, most people like and in fact crave the food they are intolerant to! Wheat products, such as bread and cakes, and dairy products, such as ice-cream, are the most common allergens and a shift away from them can result in a 'quick-win' water and fat loss of 1.5 to 3kg (3 to 7lbs).

You may find that the increase in energy and decrease in weight is so enjoyable that you don't want to go back to eating the foods which your body can't tolerate. However, re-introducing the foods after a reasonable length of time, say three months, is often fine, as long as they are not eaten in excess.

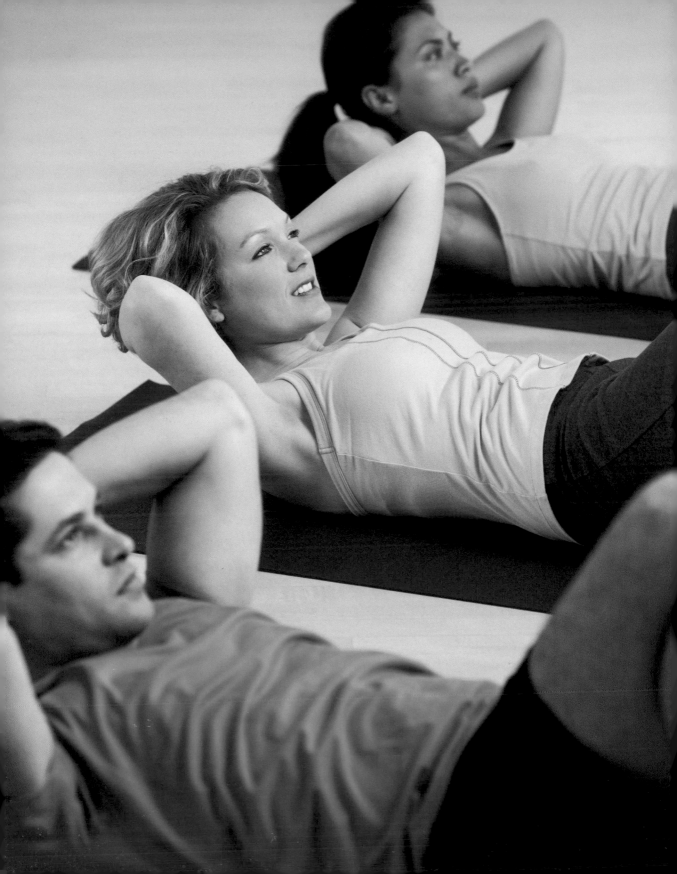

The importance of exercise

The final piece of the life-changing weight loss picture is exercise. Human beings are designed to move and you can't expect your body to perform as you would like it to without taking this into consideration. If your only exercise is stretching to reach the remote control, then tuning into your body's needs is going to be impossible.

Exercise is not only great for weight loss, but it's vital for preventing serious health problems. Even though your focus may be firmly on shifting the kilos, the life-changing plan also helps prevent health problems developing on all levels. A lack of exercise predisposes the body to harmful cholesterol and increases the risk of heart disease. A regular exercise programme can also build good bone density and boost digestion. Given that an estimated one in five adults suffer from some sort of digestive complaint, and one in three women and one in 12 men over the age of 50 will fracture a hip, wrist or spine as a result of osteoporosis, it is worthwhile taking exercise seriously.

Even more worrying is some recent research from the US, which studied the impact of lack of exercise on contracting cancer. Researchers looked at what led to the deadly disease in the first place. Although most diseases have multiple causes, the scientists were able to estimate how much factors such as infections, eating, drinking or smoking contributed. The research, which was published in the *Journal of the American Medical Association*, estimated that about one-third of all cancer deaths in the US are related to smoking, but about another third are linked to nutrition, excess weight and physical inactivity. For the majority of Americans who do not smoke, dietary choices and physical activity are the most important factors in determining their cancer risk.

Not only does a lack of exercise affect you physically, but it has a mental impact too. It is one of the undisputed facts in modern medicine that exercise is a safe, effective and vital component of being happy. Why happy? Well, endorphins, the chemical messengers that are released when you exercise, help you to feel happier, and exercise is a well known antidote to stress, anxiety and mild depression.

Cellulite can be improved with exercise, too. Your lymphatic system, which is your body's waste disposal unit, depends on movement to help it carry waste from the body. A lack of exercise can cause this lymph to become stagnant and congested, and one sign of this is cellulite. Exercise and, although it may not go away altogether, your cellulite should look better.

Losing weight alone doesn't tone or strengthen the body. It doesn't give you more stamina to live life to the full. Only exercise can do this, but if you have a sedentary lifestyle, even a gentle introduction to exercise will boost your weight loss programme, as well as delivering these other benefits.

Surprising as it may seem, exercise can really help curb appetite in those with a tendency to overeat. Most people think that exercise will increase the amount you eat, but surprisingly the opposite is the case, since aerobic exercise increases glucose and fatty acids in the blood by stimulating tissues to release their energy stores.

In terms of weight loss, the main benefit of exercise is that it really helps keep weight off in the long term. As you build lean muscle mass your resting metabolic rate, which determines how slowly or quickly your body uses energy and thus burns calories, can increase. This means that your body starts to burn more calories, even when you are resting.

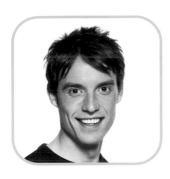

For the mind: Uncover the beliefs and emotions that prevent weight loss

Take a moment to tune into your mind and register what you're thinking about, whether it's a meeting you've got later, some shopping you need to do or something you watched on TV last night. The thoughts you are aware of exist in what's called your conscious mind, but you also have an unconscious mind, which you aren't aware of during your day-to-day life.

Your unconscious mind performs many remarkable tasks. It helps you make sense of life events, stores your memories, drives your habits and behaviours, creates your emotions and heals your body. Knowing how your unconscious mind interacts with your body enables you to harness its power to create the body you want.

Your unconscious mind is linked to your autonomic nervous system, which regulates your heartbeat, blood pressure, digestion and metabolism, along with many other bodily functions. Because of this connection, whatever your mind believes, perceives and experiences can potentially be communicated to the rest of your body, causing a physical response.

Your mind also impacts on your body through your emotions. When you experience an emotion, chemical signals are released into your bloodstream. These communicate with individual cells and have the power to affect your whole body. Immediate mind–body connection responses include getting a red face when you're embarrassed or your mouth watering when you think of a food you love.

Gradual weight gain is a subtle example of the mind–body connection, but by discovering its hidden mental and emotional causes you can more easily create and enjoy the body you want, for life.

Beliefs shape your body

Your beliefs are the conclusions you've come to about yourself, including your body, other people and the world you live in. Your beliefs exist in your unconscious mind, automatically guiding you through your life. They help you to make sense of and respond to the events and environments you encounter. Most of your beliefs are formed by the age of six, which is incredible considering how much they can impact on your body for the rest of your life.

Your beliefs determine the messages that are sent from your brain to your body. Amazingly, it has been found that your beliefs have the power to influence every aspect of your physical functioning, including your digestion, immune system, blood pressure and even your DNA. In a very real way, your beliefs become your biology.

In one scientific study, patients were given morphine for serious pain for three days and on the fourth day the morphine was secretly swapped for a simple saltwater solution. However, despite not receiving any morphine whatsoever, the patients experienced the same levels of pain relief as they had during the previous three days. The patients' belief alone had stopped the pain.

There have also been well documented cases of people with multiple personalities in which one of the personalities believed he or she had perfect eyesight and another believed that he or she was almost blind without glasses. In such cases, the personality that was dominant at any given time determined how well the person's eyes worked. The same has also been found in other cases, where one personality believes he or she is allergic to oranges, but the other personality can drink orange juice without any adverse physical effects.

Apparent miracles like these are possible because your body is designed to follow the orders given to it by your brain. Your brain interprets the external environment based on your beliefs, and then tells your individual cells what adjustments they need to make in order to survive in that environment.

The implications of this are massive when it comes to taking charge of the shape and weight of your body. If you want to change your body you need to discover and change the beliefs that are causing your body to be its current size. For instance, if you believe you cannot lose weight easily then your brain will order your body to store weight. Or if you believe thin people get ill more easily, then your mind, which is designed to preserve your body, will do everything in its power to keep you healthy by holding on to that extra weight.

Below is a list of 'body beliefs'. Write out those that apply to you and score that belief out of ten, depending on how strongly you believe it.

Body Beliefs

- I cannot lose weight easily
- It is impossible for me to lose weight
- I am big boned
- I have a slow metabolism
- If I eat too much I will get fat
- It is natural to put weight on as I get older
- Fat people have more fun
- I am this weight naturally
- I need someone to love and accept me as I am before I can lose weight
- I will not be loved if I am thin
- I will put it all back on again
- Thin people get ill more easily
- My family and/or friends are overweight, so it's natural that I am too
- People love me the way I am
- My body is broken
- Staying slim is boring
- Losing weight requires hard work
- I've always been overweight – it's just the way I am
- I eat when I am bored
- I feel guilty every time I eat
- I eat when I am anxious
- I eat when I am.....................
- I have been told I'm fat by .... for...........................years

You'll know if a belief applies to you, because you'll get an emotional response when you read it and it will feel true. You'll probably also see a connection between that particular belief and how you tend to feel and behave during your day-to-day life. Feel free to add any other beliefs you have about your body. I'll show you how to change your body beliefs in Step 2 (see page 70).

Stress slows slimming

One of the key ways in which your beliefs impact on your body is through stress. It has been suggested that 90 per cent of all disease is caused by stress and 100 per cent of all stress is caused by 'bad' beliefs.

Have you ever noticed how one person can respond to an event, whether it's giving a presentation or experiencing a flight delay, by getting very stressed, while another takes exactly the same event in their stride? The fundamental difference between how the two people respond to a potentially stressful situation is their beliefs.

If your beliefs are causing you to interpret life events in such a way that you are stressed, then your mind and body is continually operating in fight or flight mode. As a direct consequence, your hunger, thirst, digestion and decision-making capabilities will all be compromised. Even your individual cells will be in protection mode by reducing their intake of protein and holding onto toxins.

In order to protect itself from the excess toxins, the body stores them in safe places, away from the essential organs, and that means in joints and fat cells. This is why living in a perpetual state of fight or flight can lead to weight gain.

To lose weight, you need to get your body out of fight or flight mode into rest and digest mode (this is when it is calm and functioning normally), but the great news is that you can reduce your levels of stress without having to change the way you live. All you have to do is change the beliefs that are causing your stressed responses to life.

Stress Beliefs

- I'm not safe
- People always take advantage of me
- I must be perfect to be loved
- Something bad will happen
- People must think well of me
- I must be in control
- People are untrustworthy
- I can't do it
- I'm not capable
- I'm bad
- The world is a dangerous place
- I'm not loveable
- Something must change for me to be OK
- I'm hopeless
- I'm worthless
- Life is hopeless
- I'm in this world on my own
- I must take care of others first
- I'm stupid
- It's going to go wrong
- I'm going to get in trouble
- I'm not allowed to be happy
- I'm unforgivable

Above is a list of 'stress beliefs'. Write out those that apply to you and score that belief out of ten, depending on how strongly you believe it. You'll know if a belief applies to you, because you'll get an emotional response when you read it and it will feel true. You'll probably also see a connection between that particular belief and how you tend to feel and behave during your day-to-day life. Feel free to add any other beliefs you have about your body. I'll show you how to change your stress beliefs in Step 2 (see page 70).

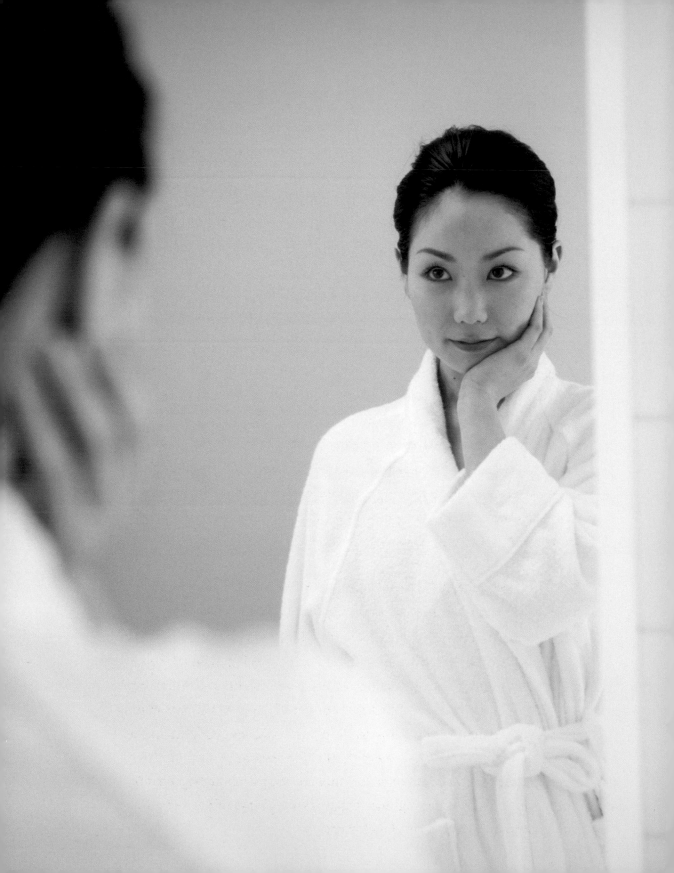

Your existing self-image

If won't surprise you to learn that the image you have of yourself can have a major impact on your mood. This was illustrated very clearly in one study, in which normal weight individuals were split into three groups, 'under', 'average' or 'overweight', according to a fictional height–weight chart. The researchers found the normal weight people allocated to the overweight group showed an increase in depression and a decrease in self-esteem compared with the people in the other two weight groups, even though in reality their weight was normal.

This fascinating research shows that it's important not to base your self-image on the opinions of others and to make sure you have a positive and loving self-image. To assess your existing self-image, imagine you are completely naked, standing in front of a full-length mirror. How do you feel about your body? What words might you use to describe its shape, weight, size and overall look? And what words might you use to describe the type of person you are? Be ruthlessly honest with yourself. Take a piece of paper or a notebook and write down the first words or phrases that come to mind, avoiding editing your thoughts between your head and your hand. I'll show you how to slim your self-image in Step 2 (see page 69).

Excess emotional baggage

Numerous studies have investigated the link between emotions and weight gain. In one particularly intriguing piece of research investigating the relationship between mood and food consumption, women were shown a sad movie to test whether it would impact on how much they ate. Amazingly, it was found that the women who felt sad after watching the movie ate significantly more food than the women who watched a movie that caused no negative emotions. This isn't to say sad movies make people gain weight, but rather that emotions can be triggers for eating more. However, it highlights that taking charge of your emotions is crucial to enjoying weight loss for life.

Your unconscious mind stores memories with unresolved negative emotions and presents them to your conscious mind for resolution at a time when you're quiet and mellow. This can cause you to feel more emotional when you're on your own without much to do.

To avoid having to deal with their emotions, it is common for people to keep themselves busy by 'comfort eating'. Common emotions to suppress with food include sadness, loneliness, boredom, guilt, worry and grief. If you know that you tend to stuff down your feelings with food, then you really can do something about this by resolving your emotional baggage and getting rid of the unconscious triggers that make you eat in excess.

Identify your negative emotions

Start by identifying your own negative emotions. In a notebook, write down on a scale of 0 to 10 (with 0 being 'never' and 10 being 'always') how often you feel the following negative emotions. Feel free to add your own as well. Rate the emotional intensity of the negative emotions you feel as well (with 0 being 'no intensity' and 10 being 'very high emotional intensity'). Finally, think about the reasons why you tend to feel how to do. I'll show you how to resolve your negative emotions in step 2 (see page 71).

• Anger	• Fear	• Grief	• Hurt	• Loneliness
• Sadness	• Guilt	• Anxiety	• Boredom	

Uncover unresolved emotional events

Significant emotional events can trigger weight gain. By significant it doesn't necessarily have to be a traumatic event in the eyes of society, the media or your family or friends. What matters is whether it was a significant event for *you*. For instance, your best friend moving away when you were six may have been a massively significant event for you, but not necessarily in the eyes of your parents.

To discover if there are any emotional issues that are linked with changes in your body shape and weight, reproduce the chart below in a notebook and plot the positive and negative events that have happened during your life. The scale on the left-hand side is the level of emotional intensity you *still feel now* about the particular event in your life (10 is a 'very positive' memory and -10 is a 'very bad' one with high levels of negative emotion associated with it).

Emotional Intensity														
10														
9														
8														
7														
6														
5														
4														
3														
2														
1														
Age	5	10	15	20	25	30	35	40	45	50	55	60	65
-1														
-2														
-3														
-4														
-5														
-6														
-7														
-8														
-9														
-10														

Having tracked the traumatic events in your life, did your weight change at around the same time as any of them? Again, I'll show you how to resolve significant emotional events that triggered weight gain in Step 2.

Find the emotional root-cause reasons for weight gain

Did you know you have a perfect memory? What you don't necessarily have is a perfect recall of your perfect memory. Your unconscious mind has a perfect record of everything that has happened during your life. This means that your unconscious mind knows why you started gaining weight in the first place. By asking the right questions you can discover the emotional root-cause reasons for your weight gain.

To help you discover the root-cause reason(s) for your weight gain, I would like you to answer a few questions. To get the best results you need to trust the first answer that comes into your mind. You don't need to know how or why you know what you do, just trust the process.

However – and this is important – if you think you could hit upon a highly emotional event then I recommend that you first learn the emotional freedom technique (EFT), so you can immediately deal with any emotion that might come up (see page 77 for more on EFT). Alternatively, you may want to seek the assistance of a trained complementary therapist (see page 157).

Ready? Let's begin. In your notebook answer the following questions.

Find the first event
• Trust your first answer – what was the first event in your life that caused the weight gain?
• Roughly what age were you?

Clarify the context
• When you think of that time, who is the first person that comes to mind and why?

- The first place and why?
- The first event and why?
- The first thing and why? Trust your first thoughts.
- Why do you think this person, place, event or thing has come to mind now?
- What might have happened that could have been a problem for you?

Identify why it was a problem
- What is it about what happened that was a problem for you?
- How did it make you feel?
- Why did you feel that way?

Try to summarise why it was a problem for you in one short sentence that includes what you felt and why you felt it. For example, 'I felt sad, scared and vulnerable on my own' or 'I felt hurt and rejected by my family.' This is the root-cause reason for your weight gain.

Once you have the statement, rate it from 0 to 10 (with 0 being 'no intensity' and 10 being 'very high emotional intensity'). A root-cause reason tends to be an 8, 9 or 10 out of 10. I'll show you how to reduce the emotional significance of that root-cause reason and bring its score down to 0 out of 10 in Step 2.

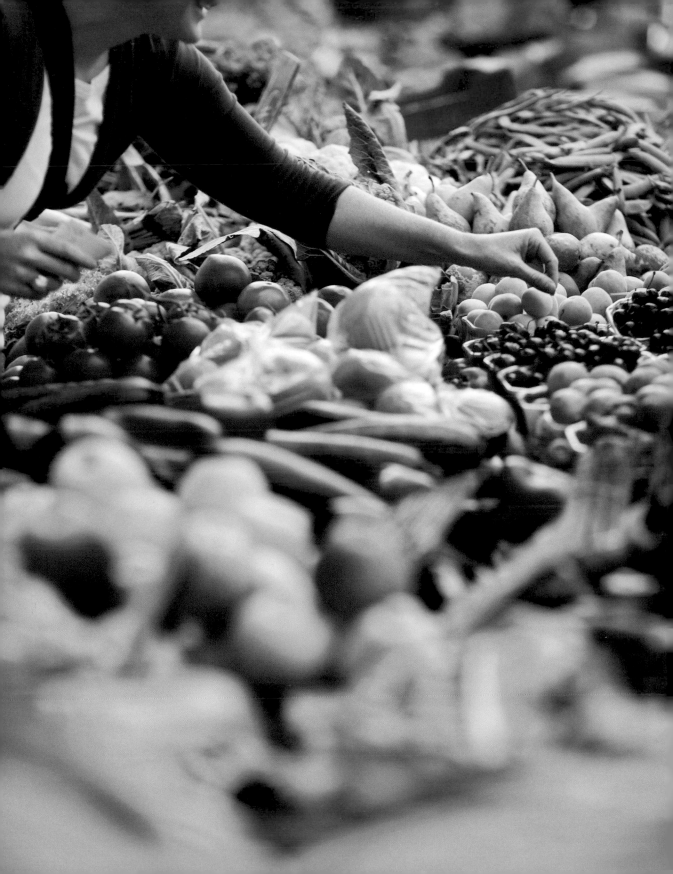

Step 2: Resolve

the reasons for your weight gain

We have repeatedly found that when our clients resolve the reasons why they weigh what they do, their weight has no alternative but to disappear, for good. Now you've discovered the physical and emotional reasons for your weight gain, it's time for you to resolve those reasons and lose that excess weight. Step 2 will help you do that.

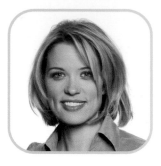

For the body: maximise nutrients, minimise weight

Ditch the diets! Forget calorie counting or complicated GI tables and start nutrient maxing now! To maximise your nutrients you need to make sure that the majority of what you consume is of the highest nutritional quality. The fastest way to ensure that these days is to go organic, but at the same time you need to stop eating fake food and start eating real food, so get rid of the processed 'nutrient robbers'. In their place, eat natural wholefoods, small amounts of protein and some essential fats, all of which are tasty and easy to use – the perfect lifelong eating programme.

The recipes in this book have been designed to maximise nutrients while ensuring that your taste buds are well catered for. You'll need to cook more than you probably do at the moment, until you get used to the system, so at the outset you should set aside time to try out new recipes, but once you're up and running you can batch-cook once or twice a week and freeze portions for future use.

Chemical clearout

If your liver can't cope with the level of toxins entering your body then your body stores toxins in fat cells. The more toxic you are, the more your body has to store, so it's time for a chemical clearout! The life-changing weight loss plan is full of nutrient-rich foods that help boost your digestion and your liver, which in turn helps your system to rid itself of stored toxic waste, but you also need to take some small positive actions in terms of what you buy and the products you use.

Dump the processed foods

Don't consume food or drink that contains artificial sweeteners, colourings, flavourings or preservatives. This is fake food that the body doesn't recognise and so it treats it as toxic. Instead, whether it's meat, vegetables or grains, choose organic food, which is more likely to be free from pesticides and harmful additives. Organic produce is also cultivated according to principles that ensure it contains more vitamins and minerals than non-organically farmed food, and it tends to be less fatty.

Avoid chemical fats

Read the label on packaged foods and if they mention hydrogenated fats don't eat them. Some cheap processed foods contain this type of fat, because it is less expensive. Trans-fats, the dangerous by-product of the chemical process used to create hydrogenated fats, are found in most processed foods yet some countries are banning their use, because they're thought to promote both cancer and heart disease.

Drink more pure water

Water helps your body to release toxic waste, so take steps to ensure you get the best quality water possible. At the very least, go for a jug filter, but if possible install a water-purification system in your home. Bottled water is a good option, but try to buy it in glass bottles, because plastic packaging is more likely to release chemicals into the liquid. Carbonated drinks, including water, contain carbon dioxide, which tends to leach calcium from the reserves in your body, so avoid them.

Go alternative at home

Try to store foods in glass or ceramic containers, rather than plastic boxes or plastic film, as food can absorb chemicals from the plastic it's stored in. Cooking equipment should be stainless steel or ceramic if possible. Avoid using conventional household cleaners and opt for natural brands instead (see Resources, page 156). If you have chemical air fresheners, throw them out and open the window instead. When in the garden, avoid the use of pesticides and insecticides.

Don't make yourself beautifully toxic!

Traditional beauty products, such as make-up, shampoo, nail varnish, hair removal creams and aftershave, all contain potential skin irritants, as well as chemicals that can be absorbed through the skin. Instead, choose natural alternatives that work (see Resources, page 156). Spray perfume on your clothes rather than directly onto your skin and use aluminium-free deodorant. Remember, perspiration is good, because it eliminates toxins, but to neutralise the unwanted smells of bacteria use natural deodorants based on essential oils. If you have to have a filling in your teeth, make sure it is porcelain (white) rather than amalgam (silver), which contains mercury, a potentially toxic heavy metal.

Stay away from the medicine cabinet

Medical drugs, although beneficial in many situations, still have to be detoxed by the liver. If you have a headache, do you pop a pill without considering whether you're dehydrated or have an underlying food intolerance? Are you taking antacids when a lack of digestive enzymes to break down your foods may be causing your heartburn, flatulence or bloating? Learn to look behind the symptoms rather than masking them with pills that add to your toxic load.

Social addictions anonymous

If you don't think you're addicted to sugar, salt, caffeine, including high-caffeine energy drinks, or alcohol, then try to go without them for a couple of days. The chances are your body will scream at you to get some quick! But here's the good news, this withdrawal effect won't last for ever and the life-changing weight loss plan is designed to help you kick social addictions that keep you overweight and unhealthy.

Say goodbye to simple carbs

Simple carbs are the danger foods of weight gain, so it's important you know how to avoid them. Remember, simple carbs are not only sugar and alcohol, and food labels may use other names to disguise them. Labels that actually use the word 'sugar', like brown sugar or sugar cane, are the most obvious 'no-nos', but also reduce your intake of foods that have any form of 'syrup' in their ingredients, such as corn syrup, high-fructose corn syrup, maple syrup and glucose syrup. And finally, look for those ingredients that end in '–ose', such as sucrose, glucose, lactose and fructose. All these ingredients are sugars and all are the enemies of weight loss.

If you find yourself in a situation where you are limited in your food options, where sugar seems to be the only choice, try to eat a form of protein with the sugar, as this will help to slow down the sugar's release into your bloodstream.

Instead of simple carbohydrates, for the life-changing weight loss plan you will eat regular small meals to keep blood sugar more balanced, thus avoiding the low blood sugar dips which lead to cravings.

Cut the caffeine

Caffeine is one of the hidden contributors to weight gain. Next time you have a caffeine hit, note your eating habits for an hour or so afterwards. Without fail, caffeine makes people eat more refined 'quick fix' foods. For life-changing weight loss, stop drinking *all* caffeine completely and switch to alternatives, such as grain-based coffees from health food shops or herbal teas. You'll also feel more hydrated, which will show in smoother skin – a nice side benefit!

Sort out your salt intake

Cutting out salt is easy when you stop eating processed foods. Remember, it's not just about the lack of nutrients in salt or the added water retention associated with salt, it's the fact that salt makes you eat more. If you want to add flavour, get creative with spices and herbs, or try a pinch of natural sea salt or Himalayan salt, which are more nutritionally balanced.

Stop smoking

Life-Changing Weight Loss is about helping you to lose weight healthily and no conversation on health can be complete without discussing the need to give up cigarettes. Tobacco has a triple toxic whammy effect on the body, from the tar, the carbon monoxide and the nicotine. If you need more motivation to give up, here are the facts on the damage cigarettes do.

Tar is a black sticky substance that settles on the mucous membranes preventing the effective removal of dust. The long-term effects of tar can be bronchitis, pulmonary emphysema, lung cancer and cancer of the throat, oesophagus or larynx.

Carbon monoxide originates from the combustion of vegetable material. It is a colourless and scentless gas. It stops the blood transporting oxygen efficiently, which in turn means the heart and other parts of the body don't get enough oxygen. It also damages the walls of blood vessels, so that fat and calcium can settle more easily. Carbon monoxide can lead to arteriosclerosis, heart complaints, cerebral infarction and brain haemorrhage.

Nicotine stimulates the nervous system, which brings up the heartbeat and contracts the small blood vessels. This causes higher blood pressure.

If you want help ditching cigarettes, then contact one of our clinics (see Resources, page 156), or find out what services your doctor offers to help you quit.

Addressing underlying medical problems
Underactive thyroid

If you think your thyroid maybe an underlying issue, start by asking your doctor to test if you have an underactive thyroid. If the result is negative and you're still getting the symptoms, then perform the Barnes temperature test – it's easy and absolutely free!

Take your temperature under your arm first thing in the morning, before you get out of bed. If possible, use an old-style mercury thermometer, but remember to shake the mercury down before you begin. Take a note of the reading and repeat the test at lunchtime. However, don't do this test if you have cold or flu symptoms as they can raise your temperature and women shouldn't do it on the first day of their period.

Two readings lower than 36.5°C, coupled with several of the signs and symptoms (see page 38), can indicate an underactive thyroid, even if it's not severe enough for a doctor to classify it as such. If you suspect you have a problem, you should see a nutritionist (see Resources, page 156).

Digestive dysfunction

If you have a digestive complaint then the life-changing plan should really help you, because it cuts out common allergens and improves the environment inside your gut. Natural probiotics, otherwise known as good bacteria, are found in onions, garlic, tomatoes, honey and bananas, all of which feature in the life-changing plan. However, it must be said that stress plays a huge part in digestion, too, so make sure you take note of the mind tools as well!

Remember, low levels of stomach acid (hydrochloric acid) affect the absorption of nutrients and you can test your levels of stomach acid with a simple home test. On an empty stomach, put a teaspoon of apple cider vinegar into a small glass of water and drink it. If you have a sensation of warmth then your stomach acid is fine. If you have no sensation in the stomach, it's because it is too alkaline and you may need some supplements to help build up the acidity and absorption, so find a nutritionist who can work on this area with you (see Resources, page 156).

Adrenal fatigue

In conventional care, adrenal testing aims to identify whether damage to the adrenals has already occurred. A nutritionist, in contrast, looks for early symptoms of adrenal fatigue when problems can be easily reversed.

I use a test that uses saliva samples to measure cortisol at several points in the day. In someone without adrenal fatigue I would expect to see their cortisol levels elevated in the morning, to help them get going, lower but steady throughout the day to sustain energy, then fall in the evening to support restful sleep.

In the early stages of adrenal dysfunction, cortisol levels are too high during the day and continue rising in the evening. In the middle stages, cortisol may rise and fall unevenly as the body struggles to balance itself, despite the disruptions of carbs, caffeine and other factors, but levels are not normal and are typically too high at night. In the advanced stages, when the adrenals are exhausted from overwork, cortisol never reaches normal levels.

If your energy flags during the day, you feel emotionally unbalanced much of the time, you sleep poorly or less than seven hours a night, you can't lose excess weight even while dieting and you use caffeine or carbohydrates as 'pick-me-ups'; these are all red flags indicating adrenal insufficiency.

The first step is to visit a nutritionist to have a full test and see where you are at on the adrenal scale. In mild to moderate cases of adrenal fatigue, significant improvement can be made through better nutrition and stress reduction alone. However, if your adrenals are truly exhausted you will need direct support through a nutritional therapy programme. The life-changing weight loss plan includes all the necessary nutrients to support your adrenals optimally, but you can also take weight-loss booster supplements for a more dramatic effect (see www.amandahamilton.co.uk for more advice on supplements). However, it is also important to reduce stress, as this is vital to overcoming the condition.

Long-term weight-loss success

Laura's story

'Every bride-to-be will understand my dilemma. It was holiday time, but with roughly four months to go until I had to order my wedding dress, every calorie was a prisoner. So I decided to do the life-changing weight loss plan and I've been eating healthily ever since, employing all the nutritional advice I picked up.

'I found it invaluable to discover that wheat doesn't really agree with me, giving me a bloated feeling, and I now only eat bread as an occasional treat. I also make sure I start the day with cleansing hot water and lemon, and a protein instead of a carb. I also have a small handful of almonds rather than the sugar and the additive-laden breakfast cereals I used to opt for. I couldn't give up on rice, but have swapped white rice for brown.

'Of course, I still have a few vices, wheat-laden pasta being one of them, but instead of tucking in two or three times a week as I used to, I now eat it perhaps once every couple of weeks. Chocolate, too, is one of my faves, but it's now organic dark chocolate instead of the poorer quality, higher-fat alternatives. Oh, and life wouldn't be worth living without the odd glass of wine – organic, of course!

'At my wedding, I not only looked, but felt great, but what's more important is I feel the plan really changed my way of looking at food. I've supersized my fat-busting ability and waved goodbye to supersized me.'

Allergies

The life-changing weight loss plan cuts out most common food allergens, including wheat, dairy, coffee, tea, citrus and lactose (the sugar in cow's milk). This will give you the best possible kick-start and should really help you lose weight. To find out if you have allergies or intolerances to over 110 common foods and drinks you can order a kit to test yourself at home (see Resources, page 156).

Effective exercise

The simple rule with exercise is to just do it! If you have a busy schedule the important thing is to prioritise it and make it part of your schedule. However, there are some 'tricks of the trade' that can help boost weight loss according to the time of day you choose to work out.

For optimum weight loss, the best time to exercise is first thing in the morning, before you have breakfast. That's when your insulin levels are at their lowest and the hormone glucagon is at its highest. This tells the body to start moving fat from our fat cells to our working muscles, meaning the calories you burn will come from fat. Your body is at is most responsive between 5 and 7pm, when your body temperature is highest and you are most flexible, so the after-work gym routine can be very rewarding. Exercising too late in the day can work against the natural body clock and can even disturb your sleep, so it's best to wind down late at night instead.

In order to make your exercise plan deliver really quick results, combine aerobic exercise with weight training, as increasing lean body mass increases the metabolic rate, therefore increasing fat loss. This means your body will be working even while you're at rest, so you can still cozy up on the sofa without feeling guilty.

In general, a minimum of 30 minutes, three times a week, is needed for your body to reflect the benefits. From this starting point you can then increase the amount of exercise you do. If you feel lost at the gym, ask for a programme or invest in a personal trainer. If you're more of an

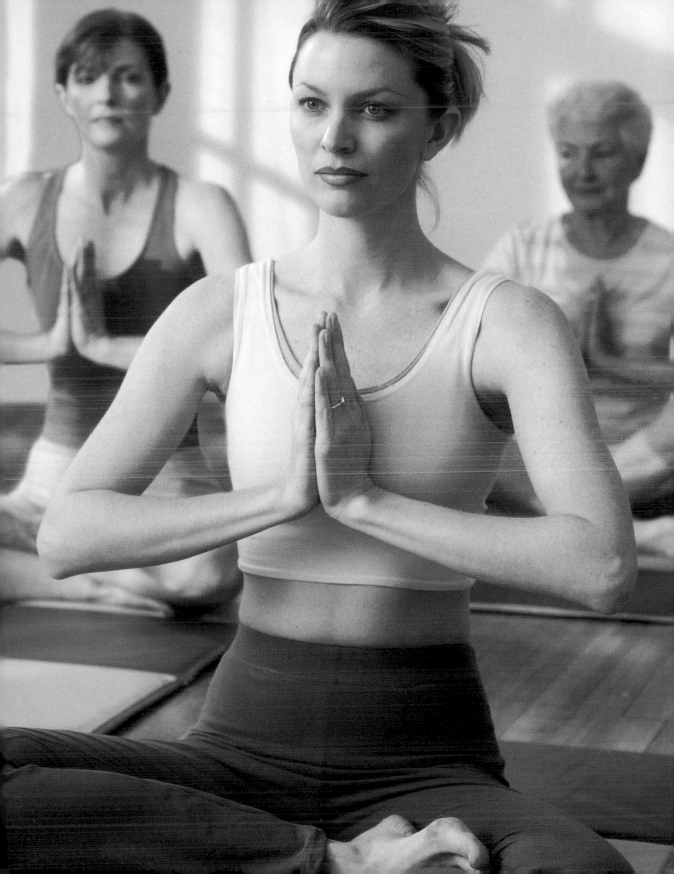

outdoors or competitive type, look for local sports clubs or activities that appeal. The most important thing is simply to have a go!

If, like most men and women, you hanker after a flat stomach, then you might want to try pilates or yoga. Both are great, not only because they deliver results fast, but also because they relieve stress. Pilates focuses on the midriff and deeper abdominal muscles to improve not only core strength but also posture – and good posture alone can give the appearance of a drop in dress or waist size. Yoga, on the other hand, doesn't focus specifically on the abdominals, but instead works with a system of 'holding in' the midriff while breathing fully throughout the session. Bizarre as it sounds, over time this system really works to tone the stomach area. Yoga has the added benefit of breathing exercises that help to calm the mind.

However, if the sound of the gym and yogic breathing has you coming out in a cold sweat, fear not, because even brisk walking will help with weight loss and has been cited as an aid to lower cholesterol and the risk of heart disease. A pedometer, a cheap little gadget that tells you how many steps you take in a day, can be really handy. If you can manage to clock up around 10 miles in a week you can lower your risk of heart disease by some 50 per cent.

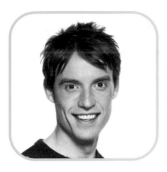

For the mind: Clear old emotions and improve your self-image

In Step 1 you established the possible mental and emotional causes of your weight gain. These included body beliefs, stress beliefs and unresolved emotional issues. Step 2 will help you overcome them. You can build a better belief system by updating your mind with the life experience and wisdom you've gathered since you first formed those beliefs, but first I recommend you focus your mind by looking again at the things you learnt about yourself in Step 1.

Improving your self-image

Remember in Step 1 you discovered your existing self-image (see page 51)? Have another look at what you wrote down. If any of the words you used were negative, here is your opportunity to create a positive statement that summarises the way to want to think and feel about yourself.

Write down the words and phrases from the lists below that resonate with what you want to be. Add your own if you want.

List A: I am a…

slim, healthy, passionate, fit, beautiful, handsome, good-looking, athletic, dynamic, powerful, slender, trim, joyful, amazing, energetic, sensational, sublime, in shape, attractive, gorgeous, strong, decisive, warm, breath-taking, dazzling, fabulous, magnificent, unique, special, lean, awesome, sexy, loving, funny, interesting, extraordinary, adventurous, creative, compassionate, energised, stunning, resourceful, exotic, patient, happy, inspiring, wealthy, genuine, kind, fulfilled, balanced, enlightened, wise…

List B: I am a...

mother, father, son, daughter, brother, sister, husband, wife, boyfriend, girlfriend, leader, winner, listener, teacher, coach, guider, lover, friend, role model, artist, entertainer, soul mate, maker of dreams, champion, angel, millionaire, dude, hero...

List C: I want to be someone who...

loves myself, inspires others, steps-up, honours myself, makes a difference, walks the talk, rocks, motivates others, respects myself, loves unconditionally, accepts others, gets results, is loved, sets new standards, shines, loves life, laughs, succeeds...

Choose a maximum of three words or phrases from each of the lists above. Put them together in the following statement, 'I am a (list A) (list B) who (list C)', for example, 'I am a slim, healthy and beautiful mother, lover and friend who loves myself and laughs.' Write down your statement in your notebook.

Say your self-image statement aloud with conviction, as though you already believe it, every day. Hold it in your mind from now on, because remember, your body is always listening! You will eventually become the person you're describing and that's what you'll see when you look in the mirror.

New, positive beliefs

In Step 1 you became aware that your body beliefs and stress beliefs have the potential to cause weight gain. From the beliefs you have already identified, pick one you want to clear from your mind now. Think about it for a few moments before writing down the answers to the following questions in your notebook. Always trust your first answers.

1. What belief would you like to change?
2. When you think about this belief, what's the earliest memory that comes to mind?

3. What emotions do you feel when you think about this memory and where in your body do you feel them?

4. At the time, what decisions did you make or what conclusions did you come to?

5. What were you deciding before then? (Keep asking yourself this question until you remember a positive belief you had decided on.)

6. If the same event happened to you today, how would you respond differently (see below)?

7. What positive effects did that event actually have on your life as a whole?

If you have difficulty answering question 5, consider what it is you now know, that if you had known it in the past, you would have never come to the negative belief in the first place. If you have trouble with question 6, ask yourself whether you are now stronger, wiser, safer and more able to love and appreciate what you have than you were before the event.

Answering questions 5, 6 and 7 often causes the negative emotions to disappear instantly, because when you think about an old problem in a new way, it's impossible to feel the same about it. This in turn causes the old belief to feel distant and be replaced with a more naturally positive conclusion. Think about what that new, positive belief might be and write it down in your book.

If your negative emotions haven't completely disappeared yet, then you can use the emotional freedom technique to help (see page 77).

Love yourself

One of the most common mental blocks to weight loss is the feeling that you're not loveable. Loving someone isn't conditional on being thinner, smarter or nicer, and that applies just as much to how you feel about yourself as how you feel about others. Believing that you're not loveable can lead to self-destructive behaviours that could prevent long-term weight loss, so it's vital that you change this belief.

To find out how much you love yourself rate the feeling on a scale of 0 to 10 (with 0 being 'no love' and 10 being 'absolute unconditional love'). If your score is less than 10, write down what you think you need to change about yourself or your life in order for you to score 10. Think about those improvements for a few moments.

OK, what you've just written down are conditions and you can cross them out immediately, because they're unnecessary. Unconditional love means love without conditions. Unconditional self-love isn't about waiting until you become someone else or have something else. The truth is you *are* loveable, you always have been and always will be, irrespective of how you look or what you do with your life. You are loveable exactly as you are now.

If this is a truth that you have difficulty accepting, you can use the following simple yet powerful exercise to convince yourself that you are loveable.

1. Stand in front of a mirror, preferably a full-length one, and while looking at yourself in it say aloud: 'I love you.'
2. Do it again, but this time take a couple deep breaths and say it more slowly: 'I – love – you.'
3. As you say it a third time, become aware of your body. Does anywhere in your body feel blocked? Do you feel any discomfort? Most people feel it in their throat, heart or stomach or the parts of their body they don't like, such as their thighs or nose, but it can be anywhere.
4. To release the resistance, say aloud: 'I love you'. Close your eyes and breathe slowly in and out through the area that's blocked. Any feeling of resistance is energy.
5. Now speak to that energy and invite it to soften and flow. It can take a minute or two for this to happen.
6. If, after a couple minutes, the blocked energy remains stuck, ask yourself what you need to learn or acknowledge for this energy to

flow. Trust your first answer and again speak to the energy block and tell it to soften and flow.

7. Now sense the direction in which the energy wants to flow – it will be up, down, to the side, backwards or straight out of the body.

8. Then ask yourself, if it could choose to leave, where would this energy exit your body. You'll get a sense of it. Whichever way it is, allow the energy to flow out of your body, reminding it gently and lovingly to soften and flow. Eventually you will sense the energy has moved out of your body.

9. Now repeat the process. This time the block may be in the same location or somewhere completely different. Repeat the process until you've released all the blockages and you can say 'I love you' and feel energised and uplifted.

10. You may find it useful to end this exercise by saying 'I love you' to every part of your body, from your feet and ankles all the way up your body to the top of your head.

A mind-changing question

Not loving yourself unconditionally causes your body stress, which is in direct conflict with your unconscious mind's desire to safeguard your body. Although not loving yourself unconditionally may provide you with some hidden benefits (for instance, by putting yourself down you get reassurance and love from those around you), it doesn't preserve the body; it hurts the body. Wouldn't it be better to let go of all conditions now and get even better results in a healthier, happier and loving way?

This question is worded in such a way that it can cause many positive changes to occur easily and effortlessly in your unconscious mind. Enjoy the results!

Helpful habits for reducing stress

Remember, stress slows slimming. For you to speed up weight loss, you need to stop your body and mind from being stressed. Here are our top three ways to reduce stress.

1. Breathe out stress

Are you conscious of your tummy? Do you tend to hold it in? Your body is designed to release stress naturally through your breathing. Unfortunately, most people don't breathe properly, which prevents the natural release of tension and places the body under unnecessary stress as it tries to operate with less oxygen than it needs.

Try this quick test. Place the palm of your hand on your stomach and breathe in deeply, noticing what happens to your belly when you breathe in. Does it go in or out when you breathe in? For most people the stomach goes in when they breathe in. However, breathing properly requires the exact opposite!

For your lungs to expand fully, the diaphragm needs to drop, causing the stomach to expand outwards. Practise breathing as you read this, making sure your stomach moves outwards when you breathe in and then inwards when you breathe out.

At the Institute of Heartmath, a US organisation that studies the link between the heart, the brain and the emotions, they've found that balancing your breathing – breathing in and out for equal amounts of time – calms the rhythms of your heart almost immediately. Smooth rhythms are less stressful for the body, helping it to rest and digest.

Try it now by focusing your attention on your heart. Breathe in for a count of five or six seconds and then breathe out for the same length of time. Do this several times. This simple exercise will help you get yourself out of fight or flight mode and will make you feel less stressed. Boost the benefits by thinking about things that make you happy. Remember, an oxygenated body and a positive mind promotes improved digestion and detoxification functioning, and therefore weight loss.

2. Rise above it all

Whenever faced with a difficult situation that has the potential to cause you stress, ask yourself what will be important about this event one year from now. Doing so can help you to rise above the details and deadlines, and instead focus on the bigger picture of what's really important.

Changing your focus can help you reduce your stress, which in turn, helps you more easily access the parts of your brain that are required for creativity and thinking outside the box. As well as enjoying better health and peace of mind, you are also more likely to get a better end result.

3. Set your stress free

If a person has done something that you believe is wrong, it's common to resist it; to argue, moan or sulk, even if you don't actually do it to their face. However, resistance places stress upon the body. Instead, make a choice to accept, rather than resist, the other person's actions. Remind yourself that everyone is doing the best they can, even when you think they aren't. Accepting the actions of others doesn't necessarily mean you have to agree with what they've done, but it does mean you've made a decision to take a more relaxed, loving and even wise view of life.

Go on a retreat

Sometimes trying to get some 'head space' in a busy life can seem almost impossible! If this is the case for you, then I recommend you treat yourself to an annual retreat. There is now an incredible array of health and well-being retreats available both in the UK and overseas, ranging from yoga and meditation to mind and body detox retreats. The right retreat can help you take well-earned time out to re-charge your batteries and reconnect with your inner peace and happiness. Sound good? Then you may want to start your search by checking out our retreats (see page 156).

Clear excess emotional baggage

In Step 1 did you discover that you have unresolved, negative emotions associated with certain people, places, events or things in your past, present or future? If so, then this is your opportunity to let go of them once and for all. By clearing your emotional baggage you will feel more at peace and be less likely to comfort eat. You will also reduce your stress levels and improve the overall functioning of your body.

Lose those negative emotions

So what if you could let go of your past emotional baggage in a much more quick and easy way than you ever thought possible? Amazing as it may seem, this is achievable due to the way in which the unconscious mind works.

Your unconscious mind is in charge of your memory and works tirelessly behind the scenes to help you recognise the people, places, events and things you encounter during your day-to-day life. Your unconscious mind does this by constantly asking, 'Where have I seen this before?' and then searches your entire mind for similar memories.

When storing memories, your unconscious mind links similar events together. For instance, angry memories are linked with other angry memories, sad memories are linked with other sad memories, and so on.

If you have negative emotions associated with past events, then, when faced with similar events today, your unconscious mind will access these old, unresolved emotions. This is why, when you hear a particular song, it can remind you of a particular place. It's also why, after a relationship break-up, it can be very difficult, because everything you do and everywhere you go ends up reminding you of that special someone, who's usually the very person you're trying to forget!

Emotionally connected memories can lead you to experience inappropriately high emotional responses to the events that happen in your life today and, as a consequence, your mind and body suffer unnecessary stress.

The great news is that because your memories are tied together with emotions you can benefit from what I call the 'emotional domino effect'. By clearing the emotion associated with the earliest memory, you can clear the emotions from all associated memories, too. This makes it possible to clear a huge amount of emotional baggage in a very short amount of time!

The emotional freedom technique

A simple, yet incredibly effective method for releasing and clearing blocked emotions, the emotional freedom technique (EFT) has been described as physiological acupuncture. It involves tapping certain points of the body, such as the collarbone (see below), which correspond with acupuncture points, while saying short phrases relating to the problem you wish to release and resolve. These short phrases are called set-up statements (you'll find lots examples on page 80).

EFT has proven successful in thousands of clinical cases and I have used it myself to help clients easily and quickly let go of all forms of negative emotions, change-limiting beliefs and even cure health conditions, such as irritable bowel syndrome, psoriasis, eczema, migraines and many more. It is often said that EFT works where nothing else will, so why not follow the instructions on the following page and give it a go? After all, you have nothing to lose.

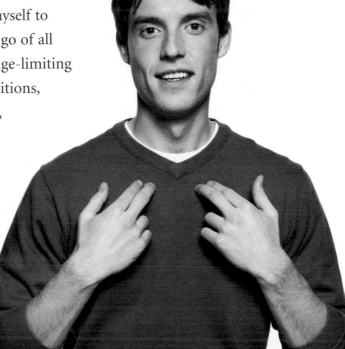

1. **Name the problem** It could be a body belief, stress belief or the root-cause reason you discovered in Step 1, but name the problem clearly, directly and truthfully, for example 'I don't believe I'm going to lose the weight' or 'I feel sad, scared and vulnerable when I'm left on my own'.

2. **Rate the emotional intensity of the problem** Use a scale of 0 to 10 (with 0 being 'no emotion' and 10 being 'extremely high emotion').

3. **The set-up statement** Repeat the problem you named in Step 1 above but add the words 'Even though' before it and 'I deeply and completely love and accept myself' after it, so for example, 'Even though I don't believe I'm going to lose the weight, I deeply and completely love and accept myself.' This is the set-up statement (you'll find more examples of typical set-up statements on page 80). Repeat the set-up statement three times while tapping the karate chop point on the side of the hand (see diagram opposite):

4. **The round of tapping** Tap seven to nine times on each of the meridian points TH, EB, SE, UE, UN, CH, CB, AP, L, TH, IF, MF, LF, KC while repeating the set-up statement at each point (see diagrams).

5. **The 9 gamut procedure** Continuously tap, rub or hold the gamut point while performing this sequence: close your eyes, open your eyes, look hard down to the right, look hard down to the left, roll your eyes one way, roll your eyes in the other direction, hum two seconds of a song you love, count up to five, hum two more seconds of a song.

6. **Repeat the round** Tap about seven to nine times on each of the meridian points (TH to KC).

7. **Re-rate the emotional intensity of the problem** Take a deep breath and measure the problem again, using the same scale of 0 to 10 (with 0 being 'no emotion' and 10 being 'extremely high emotion').

If it is higher than 0 then repeat the sequence from steps 3 to 7 using a new set-up statement: 'Even though *I still* don't believe I'm going to lose the weight, I deeply and completely love and accept myself.'

Tapping points

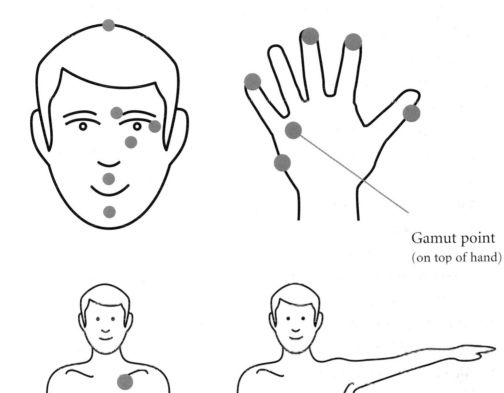

Gamut point
(on top of hand)

Key to the meridian points

TH: top of head	AP: armpit
EB: eyebrow	L: liver
SE: side of eye	TH: thumb
UE: under eye	IF: index finger
UN: under nose	MF: middle finger
CH: chin	LF: little finger
CB: collarbone	KC: karate chop point

Example set-up statements

- Even though I don't believe I'm going to lose the weight
- Even though I feel hurt about being abandoned
- Even though I feel completely empty inside
- Even though I feel anxious all the time
- Even though nobody in my family is slim
- Even though I haven't been successful losing weight in the past
- Even though I'm afraid I will still be unhappy if I lose the weight
- Even though I believe people put on weight when they get older
- Even though I have to finish what's on my plate even if I'm full
- Even though my mother's/father's words made me feel worthless
- Even though I eat because it makes me feel free and in control
- Even though I eat to numb the pain from my mother's/father's death
- Even though I feel upset about my parents' divorce
- Even though I don't deserve to reach my ideal weight
- Even though I am safer when I am overweight
- Even though I feel scared about losing the weight
- Even though I feel hurt about being abandoned
- Even though I feel sad, scared and vulnerable since my mother/father/partner left
- Even though I feel lost and alone
- Even though I feel angry/guilty/sad about what happened when I was ___ years old
- Even though I feel guilty about losing weight because my family and friends are still overweight

Long-term weight-loss success

Anna's story

From the age of three Anna had stockpiled food around the house and she had been overweight almost all her life. At 32 she openly admitted that she was a classic case of someone who knows what she *should* eat, but doesn't do it. She also recognised that she tended to comfort eat in the evenings, especially when she was alone or with close friends who wouldn't judge her.

I quickly established that one of the main root-cause reasons for her eating habits related to feeling 'hurt, sad and scared mum was so angry all the time,' which scored 10 out of 10 on emotional intensity. After just one round of tapping with EFT, this score was reduced to 0 out of 10 and she felt much more compassionate towards her mother.

I also used EFT to release the following beliefs that Anna became aware of through our discussions: 'I'm an anxious person,' 'I'm a bad person,' 'I'm sad there's always something wrong with me,' 'I shouldn't be happy' and 'I'm not allowed to be happy'.

These were all very important beliefs to clear, because they could have unconsciously driven Anna to self-sabotaging behaviours, such as binge eating, whenever she was unhappy.

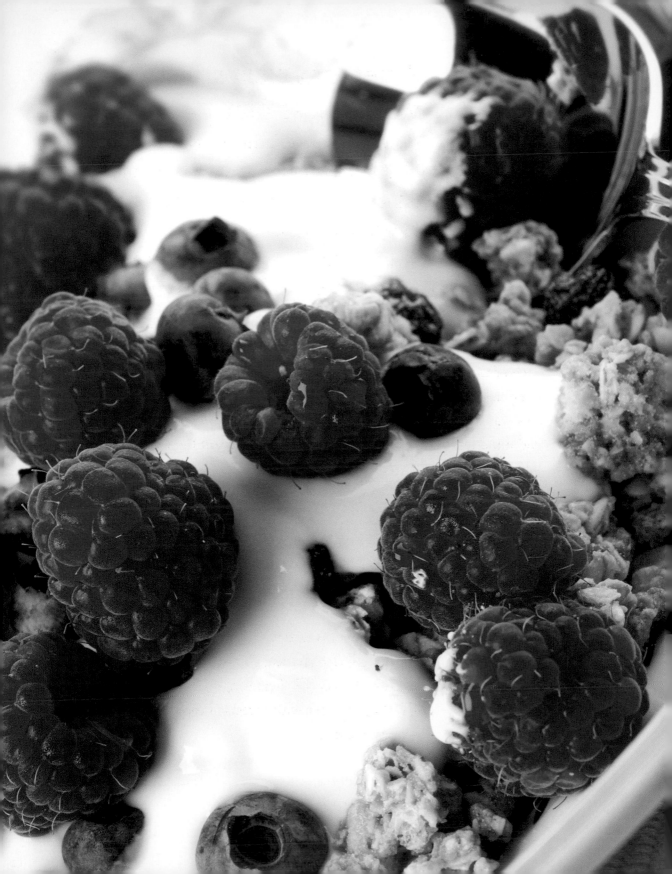

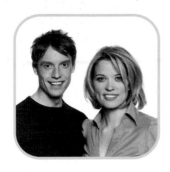

Seven-day, kick-start weight loss plan

Now that you're familiar with the various hidden ways in which your body and mind affect your ability to lose weight, hopefully you will have begun to incorporate the suggestions and exercises in this section into your diet and lifestyle. The seven-day kick- start plan is designed to help you do just that – fast.

Each of the seven days has its life-changing lesson for both body and mind, to make sure that after your first week you're able to adopt this new way of eating and thinking for the long term. You'll find the body and mind lessons on pages 83–93, while guidance on the weight-loss plan and the recipes themselves begin on page 95.

Day 1

For the body   **The Five Fundamental Food Rules**
For the mind   **Believing Before Seeing**

Menu

Breakfast: Very berry breakfast smoothie (see page 98)
Lunch: Avocado, spinach and feta cheese pancake (see page 98)
              with mixed green salad (see page 119)
Dinner: Thai chicken curry with shredded cabbage and
              coconut (see page 99)

Day 2

For the body   **Shaping up Your Body**
For the mind   **Shaping up Your Self-image**

Menu

Breakfast:	Berries with quick muesli (see page 100)
Lunch:	Carrot, lentil and coriander soup (see page 100) with rye or pumpernickel bread and rainbow salad (see page 119)
Dinner:	Mixed vegetable frittata (see page 102) with fresh herb salsa and mixed green salad (see page 119)

Day 3

For the body	**Maximise the Nutrients**
For the mind	**Minimise the Fattening Beliefs**

Menu

Breakfast:	Booster breakfast smoothie (see page 103)
Lunch:	Hearty salad with quinoa and feta cheese (see page 103)
Dinner:	Nutty fish with carrots in coconut (see page 104) and mixed green salad (see page 119)

Day 4

For the body	**Eat the Right Amount**
For the mind	**Avoid 'Eating' Your Negative Emotions**

Menu

Breakfast:	Pancake with mixed berries (see page 105)
Lunch:	Egg in a tomato cup on pumpernickel (see page 106) with sunshine salad (see page 119)
Dinner:	Thai fishcakes with salsa (see page 106) and mixed green salad (see page 119)

Day 5

For the body	**Eat Fat to Lose Fat**
For the mind	**Think Slim to be Slim**

Menu

Breakfast: Baked banana (see page 108)

Lunch: Vegetable and nut roast (see page 109) with tomato
               sauce (see page 121) and mixed green salad (see page 119)

Dinner: Tuna steak with cucumber, dill and wild rocket salsa
               (see page 110), and rainbow salad (see page 119)

Day 6

For the body   **Eliminate Physical Toxins**
For the mind   **Eliminate Emotional Toxins**

Menu

Breakfast: Pear with quick muesli (see page 111)

Lunch: Vegetarian chilli (see page 112) with brown rice and
               rainbow salad (see page 119)

Dinner: Leek, celeriac and feta frittata (see page 114) with
               mixed green salad (see page 119)

Day 7

For the body   **Energise Your Food**
For the mind   **Energise Your Life**

Menu

Breakfast: Quinoa porridge with honey
               (see page 115)

Lunch: Red lentil curry
               (see page 115)
               with brown rice and
               sprouted salad (see page 120)

Dinner: Baked sesame chicken with
               Chinese-style vegetables
               (see page 116)

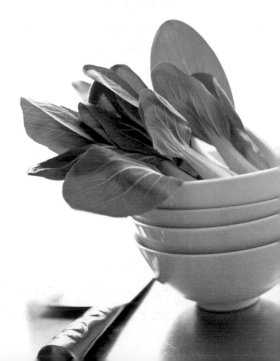

Day 1

For the body: The five fundamental food rules

This seven-day kick-start plan will keep you right on track this week, but before you begin it's important that you have grasped the five fundamental food rules, as these will serve you well in the long term.

- **Avoid eating when stressed**

  Do this by pausing and taking a breath before each bite.
- **Only eat when hungry**

  If you think you're hungry but have eaten within the last two hours, drink a glass of water instead as you're probably just dehydrated.
- **Digestion starts in the mouth**

  Chew all your food well and eat slowly.
- **Read the label even if you don't understand it**

  If you can't pronounce the names of the ingredients the chances are they're toxic! If you do buy packaged food, though, check the sell-by and use-by dates and try to make sure it is as fresh as possible.
- **Be prepared for quick meals**

  Make sure you always have a good stock of the ingredients for meals that can be put together quickly, such as stir-fries, soups and salads.

For the mind: Believing before seeing

Whether it's a smaller waist or simply increased vitality, write down what you want to achieve by following this plan. Look at what you've written and on a scale of 0 to 10 (with 0 being 'no belief' and 10 'absolute belief') how much do you believe it is possible to achieve and sustain your target?

If your belief is anything below 10, then your mind is not 100 per cent behind this project and it may be sending conflicting messages to your body. That could seriously limit your ability to lose weight, so use the techniques on pages 70 to 73 to clear your mental and emotional blocks and increase your score to 10 out of 10.

Day 2

For the body: Shaping up your body

I've already explained the importance of exercise for weight loss, but this is such an important lesson I want to remind and inspire you to get moving!

Cardiovascular exercise is one of the best health insurance policies in the world, but despite its calorie-burning and heart-protecting benefits, used alone it's not the complete method for weight loss. For toning and shaping you really need to add some resistance training. This kind of workout, using weights, machines or body-weight exercises like push-ups, has the added advantage of raising your metabolic rate, so that you burn more calories at rest, which is a huge advantage in the weight-loss game.

Of course, it's important that you enjoy what you do, but remember, sometimes we don't enjoy it until we see the results, so stick with it!

For the mind: Shaping up your self-image

Your unconscious mind will do everything it can to ensure your body and your life reflect your self-image, so check your current self-image by repeating the exercise in Step 1 (see page 51). If it's less than 100 per cent positive, have another go at improving it with the exercise in Step 2 (see page 69).

Day 3

For the body: Maximise the nutrients

Have you ever binged on lentil soup? Or over-eaten mackerel or salmon? Probably not! When the body is fed 'real' food rather than 'fake' food then we feel full and satisfied, because we've given our body what it needs to work optimally.

Remember, always *nutrient max* your meals. The recipes in *Life-Changing Weight Loss* are designed to do just that, but start to think in terms of eating what your body actually needs. For example, just a small handful of nuts and seeds as cereal and a yoghurt topping can provide most of the micro-minerals, such as zinc and selenium, that help keep cravings at bay and boost immunity.

For the mind: Minimise the fattening beliefs

Your body is designed to follow the orders it's given by your brain so what your mind believes your body becomes. Body beliefs impact on the messages that travel from your brain to your body, so check whether you have any remaining beliefs that could be negatively impacting your current shape and weight (see page 47). If you do, try the exercise that helps you achieve new, positive beliefs again (see page 70).

To lose weight you also need to get your body out of survival mode, so check whether you still have stress beliefs that are causing you to respond to life events in a stressful way (see page 49). If you have, practise breathing out the stress and rising above it all (see page 74).

Day 4

For the body: Eat the right amount

How much is enough? Obviously, the amount of food you should consume in a day depends on your body size and lifestyle. However, given that not many of us are championship boxers or whippet-like marathon runners, let's talk about averages.

An average man or woman should consume the following in a day:
• Two heaped teaspoons or one small handful of seeds and nuts
• Two tablespoons of flaxseed oil or other omega-3-rich oil
• Two servings of protein – nuts, pulses, tofu, quinoa, eggs, fish or meat

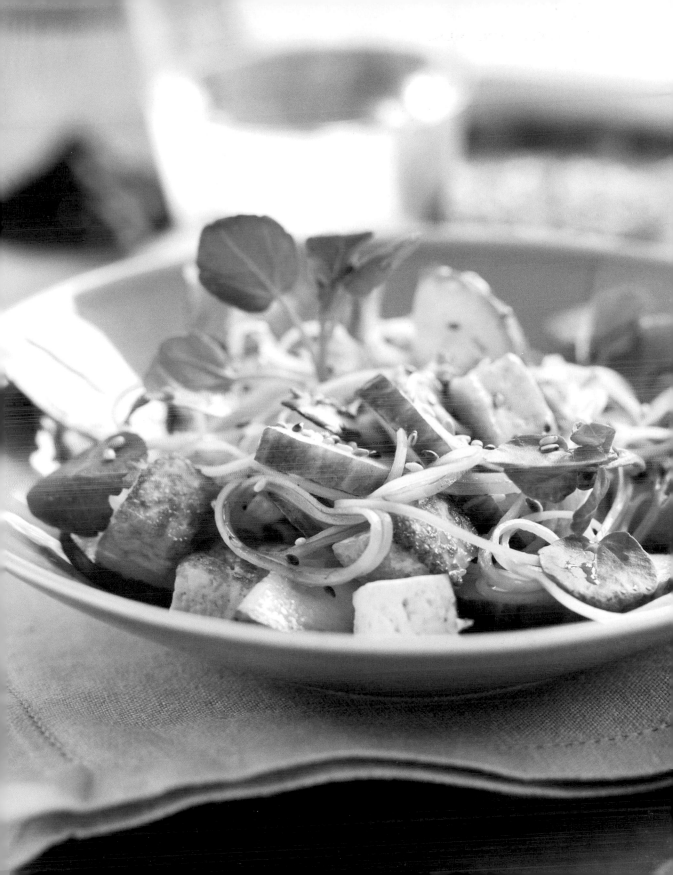

- Two to three servings of wholegrains
- Plenty of fresh fruit
- Plenty of fresh vegetables
- Two litres of fresh water plus one small glass of fresh juice if desired

Two handfuls of food at a time is usually considered more than enough and the vast majority of meals are filling and satisfying if you use nutritious ingredients and chew slowly, thus allowing the 'full' signal to get through. However, there is one delicious caveat to this rule – there is no limit to how many vegetables you can consume, so you can pile that plate as high as you want! That's because kilo for kilo, vegetables are the most nutrient-rich and low-calorie foods around.

To get maximum benefits, you should also eat a variety of fruit and vegetables, because they each contain different combinations of fibre, vitamins, minerals and other nutrients. Besides, eating the same ones every day would be boring. Good quality protein should come in portion sizes amounting to the size of your clenched fist. This doesn't mean as wide as a fist but the approximate shape on the plate.

For the mind: Avoid 'eating' your negative emotions

Feeling compelled to comfort eat can be your unconscious mind's way of pacifying unresolved negative emotions. If you feel this is one of your behavioural patterns, have another go at discovering the root-cause reasons for your weight gain (see page 54) and then do some more work on resolving them (see page 76).

Day 5

For the body: Eat fat to lose fat

Fat is actually a vital nutrient and is an important part of your diet, because it supplies the essential fatty acids needed for vitamin absorption, healthy skin, growth and the regulation of bodily functions. In fact, eating too little fat can actually cause a number of health problems. The right kinds of fat, in the right amounts, can also help you to feel fuller for longer, so try not to think of fat as your mortal diet enemy, but rather a useful ally in the pursuit of your healthier lifestyle!

Add a little fat to your meals to help your body absorb nutrients and enhance the flavour of your food, but choose the healthy fats found in avocados, oily fish, nuts, seeds, flaxseed oil and extra virgin olive oil. The omega-3, -6 and 9 fats from these foods are called 'essential' because your body can't make them itself. Saturated fats from animal products and coconut should only be eaten in moderation, while the hydrogenated fats found in processed foods should be completely eliminated.

For the mind: Think slim to be slim

Remember, your body is always listening and responding to the messages sent to it from your mind! By now you're probably some way to an improved self-image and you hopefully have some new beliefs about your body. However, one of the most common mental blocks to weight loss is the belief that you are not loveable. This just isn't true, so celebrate your worth as a human being and do the 'I love you' exercise again (see page 72). It would also be helpful to do the 'feelingisation' exercise described on page 135.

Day 6

For the body: Eliminate physical toxins

The life-changing weight loss plan is full of foods that will help clear out excess toxins from your body, but you can also boost your body's detox capabilities by working up a sweat! Exercise is wonderful, but for those days when you need to wind down, having a sauna is a great way to promote toxic elimination and also relieve stress. A sauna leaves the body refreshed and rejuvenated – just make sure you drink plenty of still water before and after the sauna (see Resources, page 157).

For the mind: Eliminate emotional toxins

By using the powerful process called the emotional freedom technique (see page 77) you can stop carrying around your excess emotional baggage once and for all and eliminate your emotional toxins. Doing so can help you feel more at peace. You will be less likely to comfort eat, your stress levels will fall and you will improve the overall functioning of your body.

Day 7

For the body: Energise your food

When it comes to bringing the weight loss plan together, learning how to prepare food in line with life-changing principles is important. However, sometimes *not* cooking is the best approach, because raw vegetables and fruits supply your body with an abundance of nutrients and enzymes, some of which are lost through cooking.

Not all you eat can, or even should, be raw, though, but try to use methods such as steaming and baking, which preserve nutrients better. Cook vegetables in a tiny bit of cold-pressed vegetable oil, adding a little water if needed, and take them off the heat when they're at the crunchy stage, so that they look and taste better, and retain more nutrients.

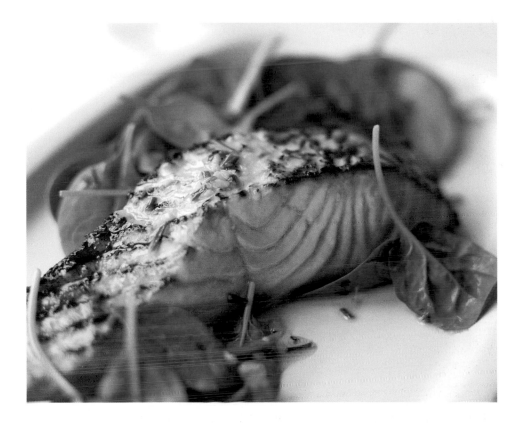

Grilling is the best high-flavour and low-fat cooking method – grilled vegetables taste sweeter and grilled meats and seafood more succulent. Frying should be avoided where possible.

For the mind: Energise your life

Setting goals is good and associating your goals with positive emotions can help increase your likelihood of achieving them. However, setting goals may also highlight the gap between where you are now and where you expect to be in the future, which in turn could lead to feelings of discontentment about your current body and life. To avoid this, I encourage you to actively choose to enjoy the journey towards your goals. Once you decide to do this you'll be surprised by how energising it is.

If you feel you need further support to reduce the volume of negative emotions you experience on a day-to-day basis, try the exercise on setting your stress free once more (see page 75).

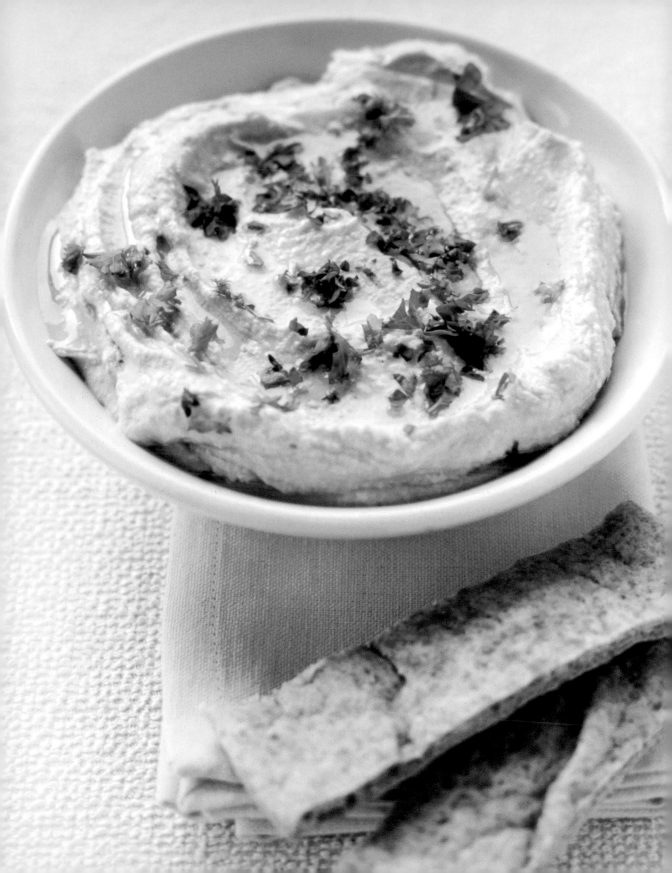

Seven-day, kick-start plan recipes

How to use the weight-loss plan

You must have breakfast, lunch and dinner each day. You should also have two or three cleansing drinks each day to boost your digestion and help your body eliminate waste. A cleansing drink is warm water with a squeeze of lemon or you can add fresh ginger if you want to.

Snack options

If you're hungry between meals, choose one of the snack options below – notice how several of them include a source of protein, such as nuts or seeds, to slow down the release of sugars. You can have a maximum of two snacks a day, but you *must* have a large glass of water first and then wait ten minutes before eating, since you may just be thirsty.

- Two celery sticks with a thin layer of nut butter (but not peanut butter) or tahini spread along them
- An apple or pear with six to eight almonds
- A handful of soft fruits with one tablespoon of natural goat's or sheep's yoghurt and one teaspoon of seeds
- Hummus with raw, chopped peppers, celery, carrot, courgette, cucumber, cauliflower or broccoli, and four almonds
- Two tablespoons of cottage cheese with raw vegetables and one teaspoon of seeds
- A hard-boiled egg with raw chopped vegetables and dressing
- A small bowl of home-made vegetable soup
- A handful of sprouted beans sprinkled with a tablespoon of mixed seeds
- An apple or pear with a slice of goat's cheese
- A rice cake with hummus
- A small pure-fruit ice lolly

• Two squares of dark chocolate
• A tablespoon of unsalted nuts and seeds (but not peanuts)
• 1 small natural liquorice bar

Daily allowances

As well as your main meals and snacks, you can have a daily allowance of the following:
• 1 tablespoon of olive oil for cooking or salad dressings
• 1 teaspoon of butter for spreading
• 2 tablespoons of flaxseed oil for salad dressings or to put in smoothies

Unusual ingredients

Most of what you need for the recipes in the seven-day, kick-start plan are available from any supermarket, but you may find you're unfamiliar with a few of the items, so here's a quick guide to some of the slightly more unusual ingredients. The majority should be available from your local health shop, but we've listed online suppliers for a few things that it may be harder to get hold of in the Resources section (see page 156). Remember, buying organic is always better if you can.

Almond milk This is a non-dairy, cholesterol-free alternative to cow's milk that's made from ground almonds.

Bragg liquid aminos This is a protein-rich liquid seasoning made from soya beans that contains a range of amino acids. Although it tastes quite salty, it has no added salt and is a healthy alternative to soy sauce.

Brown rice flour This is gluten-free flour made from whole grains of rice.

Buckwheat flour This is flour made from gluten-free buckwheat, which is actually a grass rather than a grain, that's high in calcium and protein.

Flaxseed oil This is an omega 3-rich oil also known as linseed oil, which may help stabilise blood sugar levels and protect against cancer. It should be used cold, for example in salads or drizzled over vegetables. It should not be heated.

Flaxseed powder This is flaxseed that has been ground to make it easier for your body to absorb the omega-3 and other nutrients that flaxseed is rich in. However, the best flaxseed powder is cold-milled, so look out for that on the label.

Green tea This is made from the same plant as black tea, but to make green tea the leaves are processed in a different way, which preserves many of the nutrients.

Lime leaves This fragrant, citrusy herb is often used to flavour Thai food. In fact, it doesn't come from the same tree that produces the lime fruit, but if you can't get hold of it you can substitute lime zest or lime juice.

Miso soup This nutrient-rich soup is made from fermented soya beans and can be quickly made from a sachet.

Psyllium husks This is a soluble fibre that helps your digestive system eliminate toxins more easily and can also help reduce hunger.

Pumpernickel bread This is a dark rye bread, originally from Germany, which contains less gluten than bread made from wheat.

Puy lentils These are small, dark green, slightly peppery tasting lentils that come from the Le Puy region in France, but if you can't find them you can use any green or brown lentils instead.

Quinoa This is a protein-rich seed that can be substituted for most grains, although technically it's not actually a grain itself, but the seed of a leafy, spinach-like plant.

Rice milk This is a non-dairy alternative to cow's milk that's made from ground rice. It often has added calcium.

Rye bread This is bread made from rye, a strong-tasting grain that's similar to wheat, but which contains less gluten that wheat.

Wheatgerm These are small flakes of wheat from the heart of the grain that contain, among other things, protein and vitamin E, which helps boost the metabolism.

Yeast-free, gluten-free, low salt vegetable stock cubes These are made from dried vegetables, herbs and spices, and as the name suggests they contain no yeast or gluten and very little salt.

Day 1

Breakfast: Very Berry Breakfast Smoothie

If it's easier, use frozen mixed berries. Use flaxseed powder to increase your essential fats or wheatgerm to boost your stress-busting B vitamins.

SERVES 1

120g (4oz) fresh mixed berries

1/2 banana

2 dsp flaxseed powder or 1 tbsp wheatgerm

1 cup almond, rice, oat or goat's milk

Place all the ingredients in a liquidiser, blend and serve immediately.

Lunch: Avocado, Spinach and Feta Cheese Pancake

This mixture should make eight medium pancakes and you can freeze the other six for up to a month. To use, defrost and reheat in a hot frying pan. The uncooked mixture will keep in the fridge for 24 hours.

SERVES 2

100g (3 1/2oz) buckwheat flour

1 large egg

600ml (1 pint) goat's or rice milk

600ml (1 pint) filtered or tap water

black pepper

1 tsp oil

1/2 avocado, peeled, pitted and sliced

50g (1 3/4oz) feta cheese, crumbled, or cottage cheese

4 cherry tomatoes, halved

1 handful of mixed salad leaves

fresh lemon juice

1 tbsp flaxseed oil

1. Put the flour in a mixing bowl. Make a well in the middle and add the egg. Whisk the egg into the flour, gradually add the milk and water, and mix until smooth. Add black pepper to taste.

2. Heat the oil in a frying pan or griddle. When hot, add about one-eighth of the mixture. Cook the pancake for a couple of minutes. Flip it over and cook the other side. Keep it warm while you cook a second pancake.

3. Divide the avocado, feta, tomatoes and salad leaves between the two pancakes. Add a squeeze of lemon, a drizzle of flaxseed oil and black pepper to both. Roll up and serve.

Dinner: Thai Chicken Curry with Cabbage and Coconut

The cabbage is a good alternative to rice or noodles and keeps carbohydrate levels down. You could use pak choi instead or a mixture of both.

SERVES 1

olive oil

1 organic chicken breast, skinless, cut into strips

1 portion Thai sauce (see page 120 for recipe)

1/2 cabbage, shredded

1 tbsp desiccated coconut

1. Heat a little olive oil (use a spray, so you only use a little) and gently stir-fry the chicken until browned.

2. Add the Thai sauce and cook for a further 15 to 20 minutes, until the chicken is cooked through.

3. While the chicken is cooking, steam the cabbage.

4. Serve the chicken on a bed of the cabbage and sprinkle the coconut over it.

Day 2

Breakfast: Berries with Quick Muesli

If you toast more oats than you need, they'll keep in an airtight container for a couple of weeks.

SERVES 1

1 tbsp organic jumbo oats

2 tbsp fresh mixed berries

2 tbsp natural yoghurt

2 tbsp mixed seeds (try pumpkin, sunflower and sesame seeds)

1. Toast the oats on a baking tray in a moderate oven for 5 minutes.
2. Put the berries in a bowl, add the toasted oats and organic yoghurt, and sprinkle on the mixed seeds.

Lunch: Carrot, Lentil and Coriander Soup

Serve this soup with a slice of rye or pumpernickel bread and a rainbow salad (see page 119 for recipe). This recipe makes four good servings, so freeze the rest for another day.

SERVES 4

900ml ($1^1/2$ pints) filtered water

2 yeast-free, gluten-free, low salt vegetable stock cubes

500g (1lb 2oz) organic carrots, roughly chopped

1 large red onion, roughly chopped

120g (4oz) red lentils

1 handful of coriander leaves, chopped

1. Put the water in a large pot and add the stock cubes, carrots, onions, red lentils and coriander.

2. Bring to the boil then simmer for 15 to 20 minutes, until the carrots are soft and the lentils have cooked.

3. Remove from the heat, cool for 5 minutes and blend.

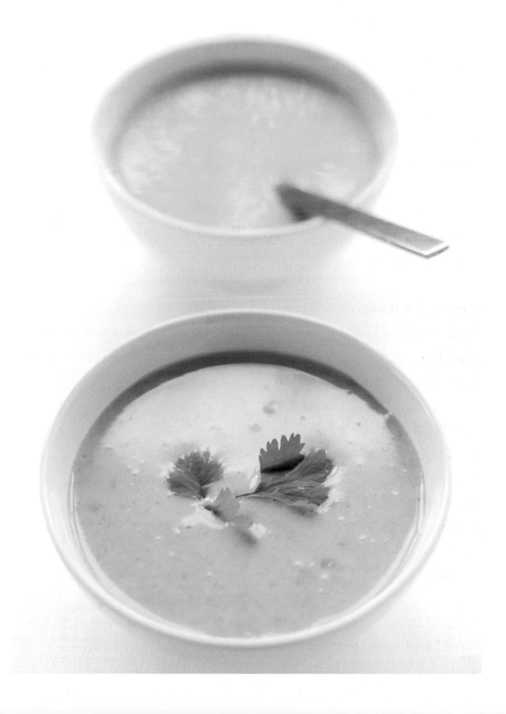

Dinner: Mixed Vegetable Frittata

Serve the frittata with some fresh herb salsa (see page 121) and a lightly dressed mixed green salad.

Use organic eggs if you can, as they're high in omega-3.

SERVES 2

olive oil

1 large onion, chopped

$1/2$ yellow or orange pepper, cored, deseeded and chopped

$1/2$ green pepper, cored, deseeded and chopped

1 large tomato, chopped

1 leek, chopped

4 eggs

2 tbsp live natural yoghurt

1 tsp mixed dried herbs

2 tbsp water

black pepper

1. Heat a little oil in a frying or omelette pan and add the onions, peppers and leeks. Cook gently until softened. Add the tomato and cook for a further three minutes.
2. Break the eggs into a bowl and add the yoghurt, dried herbs, water and the pepper to taste. Beat these together.
3. Pour the egg mixture over the vegetables in the pan and cook gently until the bottom is firm.
4. Take the pan off the heat then put it under a medium grill and cook until the top of the frittata is just brown.

Day 3

Breakfast: Booster Breakfast Smoothie

SERVES 1

120g (4oz) fresh mixed berries

1 small pear

2 dsp flaxseed powder or 1 tbsp wheatgerm

1 cup almond, rice, oat or goat's milk

Place all the ingredients in a liquidiser, blend and serve immediately.

Lunch: Hearty Salad with Quinoa and Feta Cheese

If you have any left over cooked chicken or fish you can add this in, too, and you can substitute cooked brown rice for the quinoa.

SERVES 1

lettuce or spinach leaves

selection of raw vegetables, such as carrot, radish, green pepper,
    beetroot, cucumber, sprouted beans, cabbage and broccoli, grated or
    finely chopped

55g (2oz) quinoa, cooked

55g (2oz) feta cheese, crumbled

1 tbsp flaxseed oil, walnut oil or fresh lemon juice

1 tbsp mixed seeds

1. Put a layer of lettuce or spinach in a large bowl.
2. Mix the grated vegetables, quinoa and feta together and pile on top of
    the lettuce.
3. Drizzle the oil or lemon juice over the salad and sprinkle on the
    mixed seeds.

Dinner: Nutty Fish with Carrots in Coconut

You can use salmon, tuna or any other chunky fish for this dish. As well as the carrots in coconut, serve it with a mixed green salad.

SERVES 1

120g (4oz) chopped nuts (not peanuts)

black pepper

2 tsp butter

2 tbsp coconut oil

140g (5oz) fish steak, boneless

1/2 tsp olive oil

1/2 tsp ground cardamom

2 spring onions, chopped

1/2 tsp orange rind, finely grated

250g (9oz) carrots, scrubbed and sliced

50ml (1³/4 fl oz) coconut milk

100ml (3¹/2 fl oz) water

2 tsp fresh parsley, chopped

1. Preheat the oven to 200ºC/400ºF/gas mark 6.
2. Mix the chopped nuts and the pepper and spread them out on a plate.
3. Melt the butter and coconut oil in a pan, and then remove from the heat.
4. Dip the fish in the oil and butter mix and then in the nut mixture. Press it down firmly. Put the fish aside on a lightly oiled baking sheet for a couple of minutes while you prepare the carrots.
5. Heat the olive oil and stir the cardamom, spring onions, orange rind and carrots over a medium heat for two minutes.
6. Stir in the coconut milk and water, and cook, covered, for ten minutes. Bake the fish for ten minutes, until it's cooked through.
7. Serve the fish and carrots together and sprinkle with the chopped parsley.

Day 4

Breakfast: Pancake with Mixed Berries

If you froze the pancakes left over from day one's lunch you can defrost one of those and reheat it in a hot frying pan. However, if you're making the pancakes from scratch, this mixture makes eight medium pancakes, so what you don't need you can freeze for up to a month.

SERVES 1

100g (3 $^{1}/_{2}$oz) buckwheat flour

1 large egg

600ml (1 pint) goat's or rice milk

600ml (1 pint) filtered or tap water

black pepper

1 tsp oil

1 handful of fresh mixed berries

2 tbsp natural yoghurt

1 tbsp chopped nuts (not peanuts)

1. Put the flour in a mixing bowl. Make a well in the middle and add the egg. Whisk the egg into the flour, gradually add the milk and water, and mix until smooth. Add black pepper to taste.

2. Heat the oil in a frying pan or griddle. When hot, add about one-eighth of the mixture. Cook the pancake for a couple of minutes. Flip and cook the other side.

3. Pile the berries and yoghurt onto the warm pancake, and sprinkle on the chopped nuts.

Lunch: Egg Cooked in a Tomato Cup on Pumpernickel

Serve with sunshine salad (see page 119), which is high in beta carotene.

SERVES 1

1 large tomato

1 large organic egg

$^{1}/_{2}$ tsp butter

1 slice pumpernickel bread

1. Preheat the oven to 180ºC/350ºF/gas mark 4.
2. Cut the top of the tomato off and scoop out all the flesh in the middle. Set this aside.
3. Put the butter into the bottom of the hollow tomato and then crack the egg into it.
4. Bake the tomato for 20 minutes, until the egg is cooked.
5. Toast the pumpernickel bread, spread the tomato flesh over it and top with the baked tomato and egg.

Dinner: Thai Fishcakes

Serve with some herb salsa (see page 121) and a mixed green salad, or alternatively a tamari dip. If you prefer salmon to white fish that's fine and you could substitute parsley for the coriander.

SERVES 2

200g (7oz) white fish, cut into chunks

$^{1}/_{2}$ white onion, finely chopped

2 spring onions, finely chopped

1 small green chilli, finely chopped

2cm ($^{1}/_{2}$ in) piece of fresh ginger, grated

1 garlic clove, crushed

1 tsp green curry paste

1 organic egg

2 tsp bragg liquid aminos

2 tbsp fresh coriander, chopped

2 tbsp brown rice flour

2 tsp lime juice

black pepper

1 tbsp olive oil (optional)

1. Mix the fish, white onion, spring onions, chilli, ginger, garlic, curry paste, egg, bragg liquid aminos and coriander together in a food processor, but leave some texture in the mixture.
2. Mix in the flour, lime juice and black pepper by hand.
3. Divide the mixture into eight, form each portion into a ball and slightly flatten it.
4. Steam the fishcakes in a steamer for about 10 minutes or shallow-fry them in olive oil for 8 to 10 minutes until cooked through.

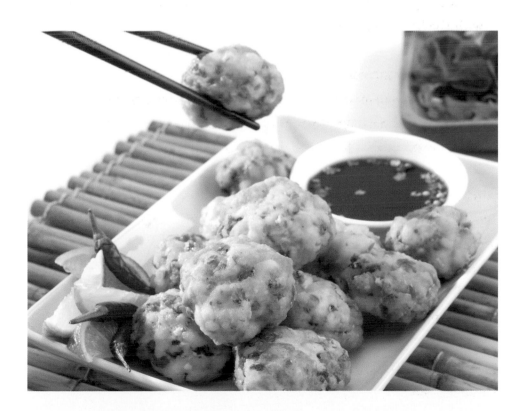

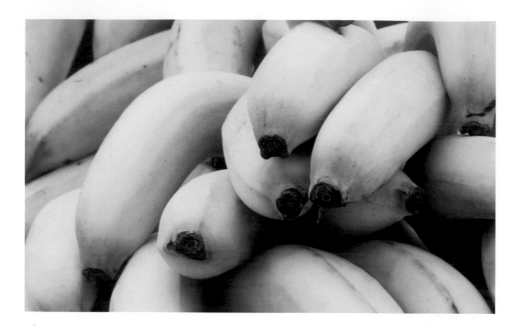

Day 5

Breakfast: Baked Banana

SERVES 1

1 small banana

2 tbsp orange juice

1 tsp maple syrup

1 tbsp chopped or flaked almonds

1 tbsp rolled oats

pinch of ground cardamom

1 tbsp desiccated coconut

1 tbsp natural yoghurt

1. Preheat the oven to 200°C/400°F/gas mark 6.
2. Peel the banana, halve it lengthways and place it on a baking dish. Combine the orange juice, maple syrup, almonds, oats and cardamom, and pour over the banana.
3. Bake for 30 minutes or until piping hot. Top with the coconut and serve with the natural yoghurt.

Lunch: Vegetable and Nut Roast

Serve this nut roast with some tomato sauce (see page 121) and a mixed green salad. It's equally good hot or cold.

Do note, though, that you should avoid having any nuts as snacks on the same day as this nut roast, as that would be overdoing the nuts.

SERVES 4

2 carrots, scrubbed

1 white onion

2 sticks celery

120g (4oz) mixed nuts (not peanuts)

4 tsp bragg liquid aminos

2 large organic eggs

1–2 tsp mixed herbs

black pepper

1–2 tbsp porridge oats

1. Preheat the oven to 190ºC/375ºF/gas mark 5.
2. Put the vegetables and nuts into a food processor and process until they're chopped into chunky pieces.
3. Put them into a bowl and mix in the bragg liquid aminos, eggs, herbs and some black pepper.
4. Line a medium-sized loaf tin with greaseproof paper and sprinkle porridge oats lightly over the bottom of it.
5. Pour in the vegetable and nut mixture, and level it down with the back of a spoon. Bake uncovered for 45 to 50 minutes.

Dinner: Tuna Steaks with Cucumber, Wild Rocket and Dill Salsa

Serve the tuna and salsa as quickly as possible, ideally while the salsa dressing is still sizzling, accompanied by a colourful rainbow salad (see page 119).

SERVES 2

¼ large cucumber, halved lengthways and diced

25g (1oz) wild rocket, chopped

1 tbsp fresh dill, chopped

2 tuna steaks

2 tbsp olive oil

1 tbsp red wine vinegar

black pepper

1. Toss the cucumber, wild rocket and dill together.
2. Heat a ridged grill pan (preferably non-stick) over a medium-high heat. Brush the tuna steaks with a little of the oil and fry them for 3 to 4 minutes each side, depending on their thickness. Don't overcook the fish.
3. Mix the rest of the oil with the vinegar and season with the pepper.
4. When the fish is done, put each steak on a warmed plate and top with a handful of the green vegetable and herb mixture.
5. With the pan still on the heat, pour in the vinegar and oil mixture, and let it sizzle for a few seconds, before pouring it over the fish and salsa.

Day 6

Breakfast: Pear with Quick Muesli

SERVES 1

1 pear, skin on, chopped

1 tbsp organic jumbo oats

2 tbsp mixed seeds

2 tbsp natural yoghurt

2 tbsp almond milk

1. Toast the oats on a baking tray in a moderate oven for five minutes (or use what you prepared on day 2).
2. Put the pear in a bowl, add the toasted oats, yoghurt and almond milk, and sprinkle on the mixed seeds.

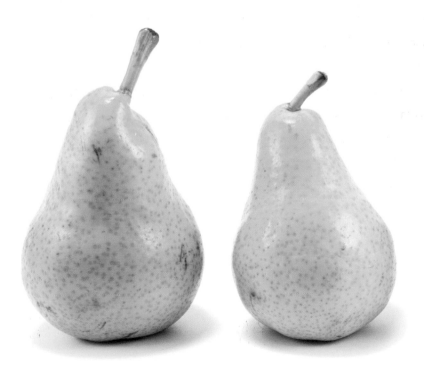

Lunch: Vegetarian Chilli

Serve brown rice and a rainbow salad (see page 119 for recipe) with this chilli. You can substitute tinned haricot or butter beans for the cannellini beans, but make sure all the beans are in water, with no added salt, and you rinse them well before use. The portions here are generous, so you may well get a third helping out of this recipe.

SERVES 2

1 tbsp olive oil

1 yellow or orange pepper, sliced

1/2 red onion, chopped finely

1/2 white onion, chopped finely

1/2 tsp each red chilli flakes, ground cinnamon, cumin seeds and thyme

2 garlic cloves, crushed

400g (14oz) tin red kidney beans

400g (14oz) tin cannellini beans

225g (8oz) Puy lentils, cooked as per instructions and drained

400g (14oz) tin tomatoes

1 tbsp tomato purée

1. Heat the oil in a pan, add the pepper and onions and cook until the onions are translucent.
2. Add all the spices and cook for a further minute.
3. Add the garlic, beans, lentils, tomatoes and tomato purée, and simmer over a low heat for 15 to 20 minutes.

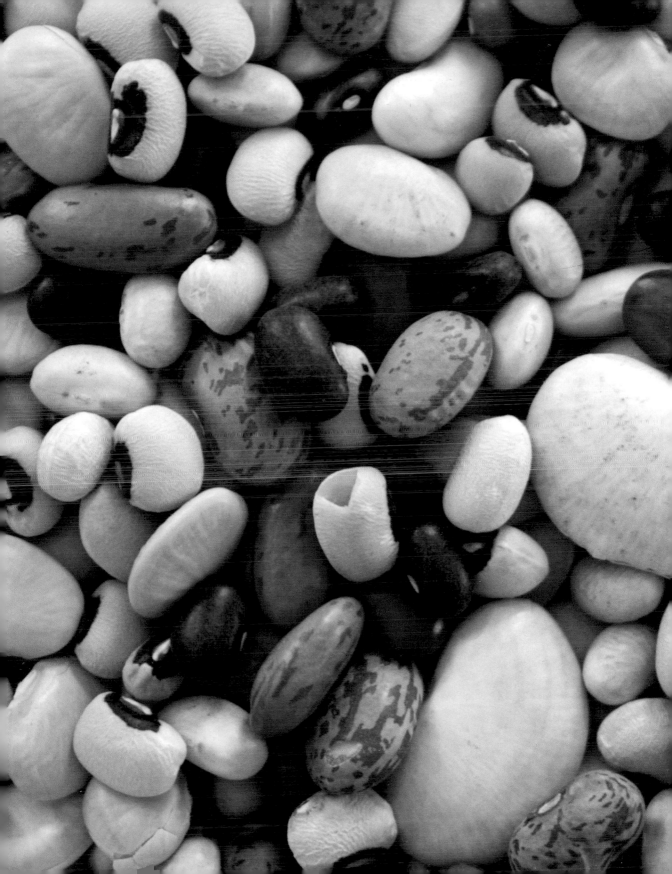

Dinner: Leek, Celeriac and Feta Frittata

Serve this frittata with a mixed green salad. It can be eaten hot or cold, so if you like you can save a portion for tomorrow's breakfast.

SERVES 4

375g (13oz) celeriac

fresh lemon juice

2 tbsp olive oil

250g (9oz) leeks, sliced

6 organic eggs

1/2 tsp mustard

4 tbsp dill, chopped

black pepper

50g (1³/4oz) Greek feta cheese

1. Peel the celeriac, chop it into big chunks and dip them in the lemon juice to stop them turning brown. Steam it for about 15 minutes until it's tender. Let it cool, grate it and then set it aside.
2. Heat the oil in a frying or omelette pan and gently fry the leeks until they're soft.
3. Crack the eggs into a bowl, add the mustard, dill and pepper, and whisk them together. Stir in the grated celeriac, feta and cooked leeks.
4. Return the mixture to the pan and smooth it down. Cook over a low setting for 10 minutes.
5. When the frittata mix begins to set around the edges, grill it for a further 10 minutes, until it's firm and slightly brown on top.

Day 7

Breakfast: Quinoa Porridge with Honey

Alternatively, if you've got a portion of frittata left over from dinner on day 6 you could have that for breakfast instead.

SERVES 1

75g (3oz) quinoa

3 tbsp soya or rice milk

pinch of cinnamon

pinch of ground nutmeg

3 tbsp natural yoghurt

1 tsp honey

1 banana or pear, chopped

1. Place the quinoa in a pan with 350ml (12fl oz) of water and bring to the boil. Simmer for 15 minutes until creamy and soft.
2. Put the quinoa, milk, cinnamon and nutmeg in a food processor and blend.
3. Pour into a bowl, spoon the yoghurt over the top, drizzle on the honey and top with the chopped fruit.

Lunch: Red Lentil Curry

The texture of brown basmati rice goes well with this curry. Serve a crunchy sprouted salad (see page 120 for recipe) with it, too.

SERVES 2

2 tsp olive oil

1 red onion, chopped

225g (8oz) red lentils

600ml (1 pint) filtered water

½ yeast-free, wheat-free, low salt vegetable stock cube

1 tsp curry powder

1 tsp chilli powder

300ml (½ pint) skimmed goat's or rice milk

1. Heat the olive oil, add the onion and cook until it's soft and translucent.
2. Add the lentils, water, stock cube, and curry and chilli powders.
3. Simmer for 10 to 15 minutes until the lentils are almost cooked, then add the milk and cook for 5 more minutes.

Dinner: Baked Sesame Chicken with Chinese-style Vegetables

If you prefer, you can use fish or tofu instead of chicken. You can also use your favourite mix of vegetables – mangetout, rocket and green beans works well too.

SERVES 2

2 chicken breasts, skinless, cut into strips

2 tbsp bragg liquid aminos

2 tsp honey

sesame seeds

1 tbsp olive oil

2 spring onions, chopped

120g (4oz) mangetout

½ red pepper, chopped

1 large carrot, chopped finely

1 bunch pak choi, chopped

55g (2oz) Chinese leaves or 2 large cabbage leaves, chopped finely

120g (4oz) beansprouts

1. Preheat the oven to 180°C/350°F/gas mark 4.
2. Marinade the sliced chicken in the bragg liquid aminos and honey for 30 minutes.

3. Roll the chicken in the sesame seeds and bake for 15 minutes.

4. Heat the olive oil in a wok or frying pan, add the spring onions and stir-fry for 1 minute.

5. Add the mangetout, pepper, carrots, pak choi and Chinese leaves, and stir-fry for 3 to 4 minutes, until the mangetout and pak choi are beginning to wilt.

6. Stir in the beansprouts and heat through for a further 3 minutes.

7. Serve the vegetables with the chicken on top.

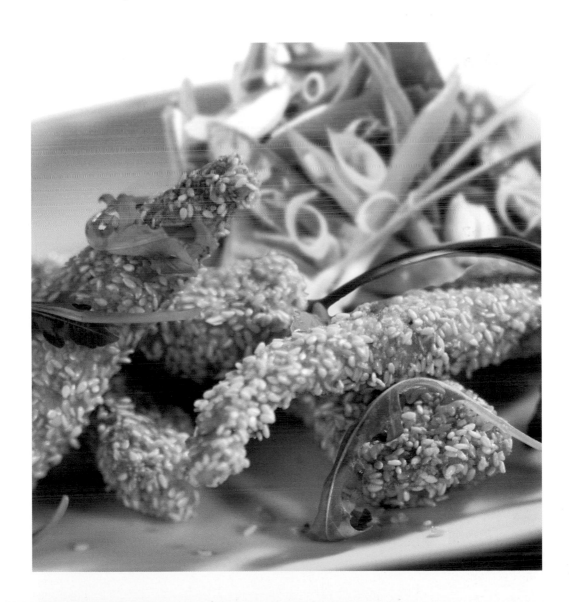

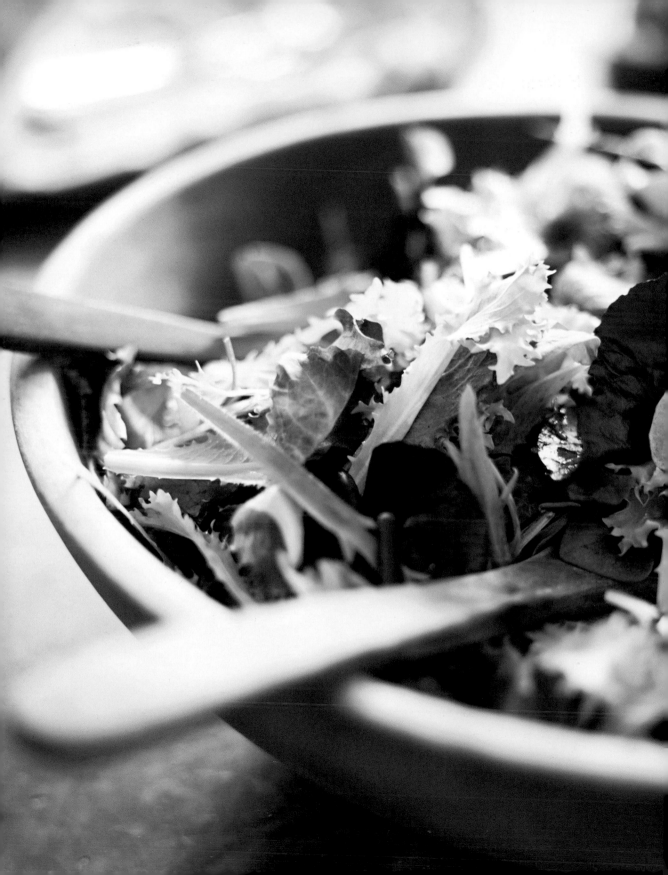

Salads

Mixed Green Salad
SERVES 1

1 handful each of wild rocket, watercress and chopped lettuce leaves

1 tbsp flaxseed oil

^{1}/$_2$ tbsp lemon juice

^{1}/$_2$ tbsp apple cider vinegar

Mix the leaves together in a bowl. Mix the oil, lemon juice and vinegar together separately and pour over the leaves.

Rainbow Salad
SERVES 1

1 large handful of salad leaves, any variety

^{1}/$_4$ red, yellow or orange pepper, deseeded and sliced thinly

^{1}/$_2$ carrot, sliced thinly

thumb-sized piece of cucumber, sliced thinly

3 cherry or plum tomatoes, halved

Mix all the ingredients together in a bowl.

Sunshine Salad
SERVES 1

2 large carrots, chopped finely

1 red, yellow or orange pepper, chopped

2 handfuls of lettuce leaves

1 tbsp flaxseed oil

Mix all the ingredients together in a bowl.

Sprouted Salad

SERVES 1

2 handfuls of sprouted beans and seeds (mung beans, alfalfa sprouts)

1 green eating apple, sliced

1 yellow pepper, sliced

1 handful of mixed herbs (parsley, coriander)

1 tbsp flaxseed oil

Mix all the ingredients together in a bowl.

Sauces

Thai Sauce

SERVES 4

4 tbsp vegetable oil

1 onion, roughly chopped

1 bunch spring onions, sliced finely

2 garlic cloves, crushed

2–3 tbsp Thai green curry paste

400g (14oz) tin coconut milk

3 tbsp fresh coriander leaves, chopped finely

4–5 lime leaves, shredded finely

2–3 tbsp fresh lime juice

a few extra coriander leaves

1. Heat the oil in a wok, add the onion, spring onions and garlic, and cook gently.
2. Stir in the Thai green curry paste.
3. Pour in the coconut milk and stir again. Bring up to simmering point.
4. Stir in the fresh coriander and lime leaves and season to taste with the lime juice. Use the extra coriander leaves for decoration.

Fresh Herb Salsa

SERVES 1

200g (7oz) tin tomatoes, diced

$^1/_2$ green pepper, diced

1 onion, diced

1 handful of fresh coriander, chopped finely

$^1/_2$ tbsp fresh tarragon, chopped finely

$^1/_2$ tbsp chilli sauce

1 tbsp cider vinegar

1. Toss together the tomatoes, pepper, onion, herbs, chilli sauce and cider vinegar in a bowl.
2. Refrigerate for at least 30 minutes.

Basic Tomato Sauce

SERVES 1

2 tsp olive oil

1 small onion, chopped

1 clove garlic, crushed

400g (14oz) tin organic tomatoes

1 tsp of mixed dried herbs

black pepper or paprika

1. Heat the olive oil in a pan, add the onion and garlic and cook gently until soft.
2. Add the chopped tomatoes, herbs and pepper or paprika and simmer for 10 to 15 minutes.

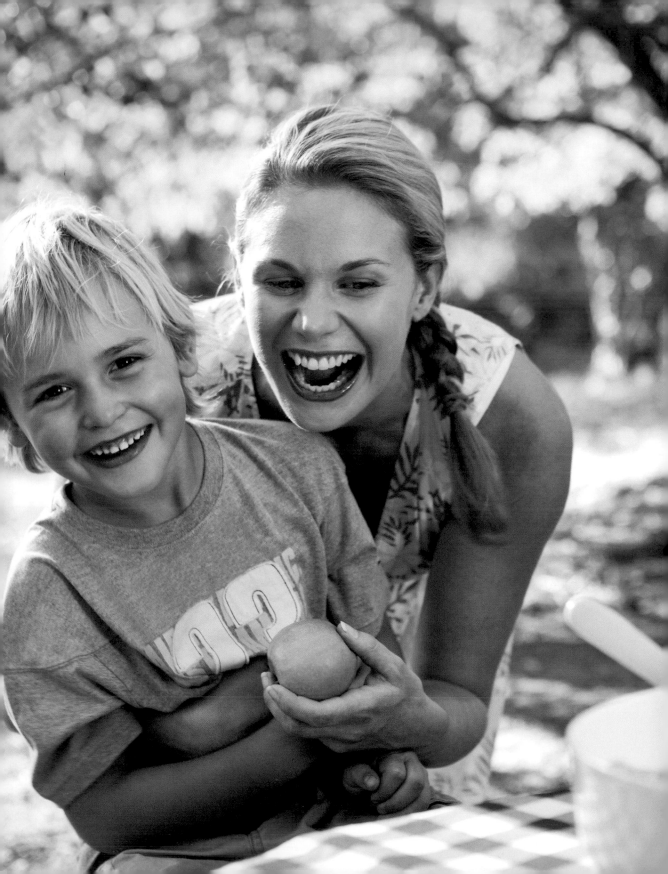

Step 3: Enjoy

the body you want for life

You've done it – you've made the decision to change your body and your life, you've shown you're committed and you've started to establish long-term eating, thinking and living habits. In Step 3 we provide some practical support, to help you continue with the plan, and show that maintaining these new habits is both easy and enjoyable.

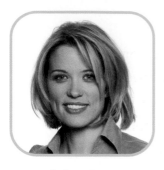

For the body: What to do next

Having completed the seven-day, kick-start plan, you are now well on the way to a new you. After this first week it's possible that your clothes may feel a little looser, but if they don't, remember that this is a life-changing plan, designed to deliver sustainable, permanent weight loss, and you're making changes that are for life.

Your true slim self may only just be beginning to emerge, but you should certainly feel full of health and vitality, as you reap the benefits of eating delicious nutrient-rich food and eliminating toxins such as sugar, salt, caffeine and processed foods from your body.

In the second week of your new life, you may feel more comfortable repeating the seven-day, kick-start plan, rather than going it alone. If you do, then that's fine, but try to mix in one or two of our additional recipes (see pages 138 to 154) and start coming up with some of your own – just make sure you put into practice the principles explained in this book and nutrient max!

As you continue with the plan, make sure you listen to what your body wants. For example, if you wake up starving, have a substantial breakfast like the ones in the kick-start plan, but if you're not particularly hungry or have to eat and go, you'll probably find a smoothie, fresh juice or a selection of fresh fruit will keep you going until you have a mid-morning snack. You can then enjoy a bigger breakfast when you're super-hungry and have more time, perhaps at the weekend, but the point is to respond to your body's needs, rather than being rigid.

Keep your balance

It may seem like it initially, but you really don't have to become a vegetarian teetotaller to get the benefits of life-changing weight loss – it's all about balance. When you eat real food with real flavour, the need for sugar, salt or processed additives is dramatically reduced and your taste buds get a chance to speak up. Fresh, natural produce is all important and none are more important than vegetables and fruits. If you've struggled to make them a big part of your diet in the past, now is the time to really make an effort. We all have days when we simply haven't got time to cook, but even then make sure you still get your portions of fruits and veg.

Vegetables are the best way to boost your nutrient intake and ensure healthy, effective weight loss. You can eat a lot of vegetables without consuming more energy than your body needs, as they're low in fat and calories. They are also a good source of dietary fibre, which helps you feel full. At least two meals a day should have half the plate covered in vegetables. If you can't manage this, vegetables can be consumed in a variety of easy ways. In order to achieve your quota, aim for the following:

• One large bowl of vegetable soup (no salt)
• One large fresh salad or two in summer (one can replace your soup)
• Cooked vegetables with your main meal
• Raw vegetables as a snack between meals

Although not as important as vegetables for weight loss, fruit is healthy, tasty and, of course, sweet. Fruit makes an ideal snack between meals and can be used in fruit salads, or in juices or smoothies. It can also be baked or stewed for delicious desserts. If you've overindulged and want to get back on track, try eating only fresh fruit until midday for a few days as it will help your body rebalance.

In terms of drinking alcohol, it's a question of balance, too. In fact, I recommend that you consume less alcohol than the UK government guidelines advise and keep it for special occasions only. Alcohol can unbalance blood sugar, making binges or cravings for sweets more likely, and it's known to increase the amount of food you consume. Wine glasses these days come in either large or goldfish bowl-size, so demand a smaller glass! You'll drink more slowly, but still feel that you're keeping up with those around you – and your liver will be enormously grateful. Another tip is to drink a glass of water between each alcoholic drink, as this will make you less desperate for the next one.

Eating out

Do you try to eat healthily, only to see all your good intentions fly out the window whenever you go out? We now live in a society where there are coffee bars on most city street corners, in stations, airports and even garages, and it's inevitable that from time to time you'll find yourself in one! In terms of coffee, the main ingredient that plays havoc with body and mind is caffeine, so go for decaf. Many outlets now serve soya milk, so if you find that a dairy-free diet suits you, switch to this option. Tea-lovers don't escape, though, since old-fashioned English tea also contains caffeine and should be cut out as much as possible. Herbal or green teas are the best option.

For an eating plan to be successful and sustainable, you need to be able to adapt it to your lifestyle, but lunch can be a tricky meal, particularly if you're out at work. Again, this is where soups are really useful, as they're available in most cafés and canteens or, better still, make your own, fill a flask and take it with you to work. Serve it with a couple of oat cakes or a slice of pumpernickel or rye bread. A big box of salad is another excellent packed lunch option. Serve it with some oat cakes, rice cakes, wholemeal or rye bread or, if you've got access to a microwave and are especially hungry, you could heat up a small jacket or sweet potato. It's also a good idea to cook extra portions of your weekend meals and take these to work.

I do recognise that the principles of *Life-changing Weight Loss* don't necessarily translate well to the average restaurant menu. However, eating plans that don't take social life into account are bound to fail – humans are social animals after all – so, as a way of bridging the gap between staying on track and enjoying a good meal out with your mates, here is a guide to what to order.

Chinese and Thai: Asian cooking is the obvious healthy choice, as it's generally high in vegetables, lightly cooked or steamed and very fresh. Fish, vegetables and tofu are the best bet, but avoid anything deep-fried and go for steamed noodles and rice instead. However, some Asian food, particularly Chinese, can include an additive called monosodium glutamate (MSG), a flavour enhancer that, in excess, can make people ill. If you eat in a Chinese restaurant, be bold and ask for it not to be included in your food. In fact, some restaurants these days advertise the fact that they cook MSG-free food.

Japanese: Japan has the highest proportion of people who have lived beyond 100 years in the world – for good reason. The basic Japanese diet is super-healthy, with lots of vegetables, including sea vegetables, which are rich in iodine and a great boost to the metabolism. Be careful of overdoing the raw fish, though, as it can harbour bacteria.

Greek, Turkish and Lebanese: Hummus, pitta bread, olives, stuffed peppers and vine leaves – cuisines like these make for veggie heaven! However, if you're a meat eater, this style of restaurant often has fresh lamb on the menu, and in a healthy proportion to the rice and vegetables.

Italian: Simple carbohydrates – think white pasta, pizza dough, bread sticks – take centre stage in Italian cooking, while vegetables and salads lurk in the background, so always try to incorporate a large salad into your meal and have a half-portion of the main meal instead. Alternatively, go against the grain and opt for the fish.

Indian: Indian food is renowned for its heavy use of oil, but if you need some spice in your life and can find a restaurant that goes easy on the

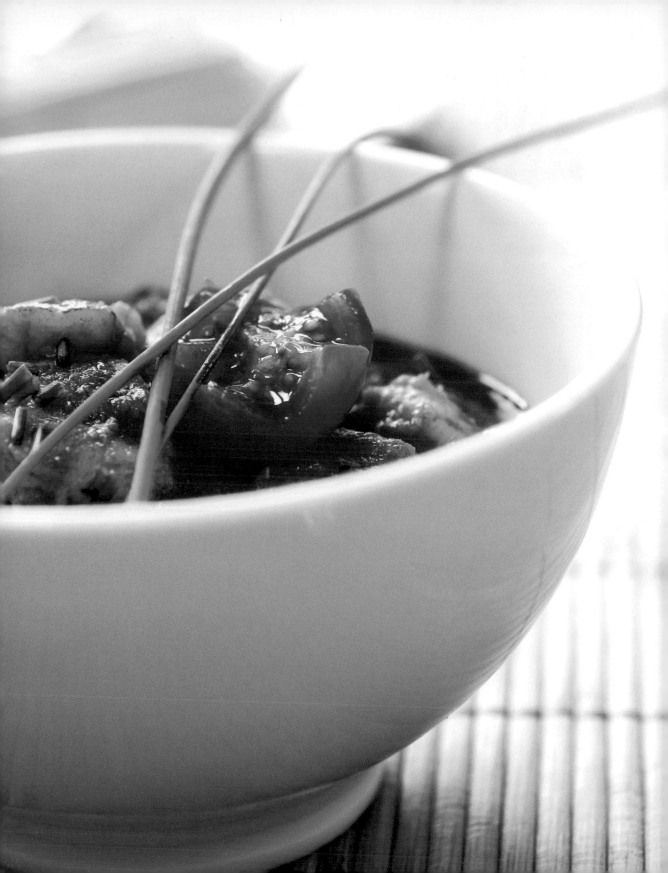

grease, at least super-healthy pulses are the mainstay of dishes such as dhal or dhansak. If you love naan bread, however, try ordering a portion of chapattis instead – they're much lower in fat and taste great.

French: French cuisine has a reputation for being rich but of course it is so much more varied than the buttery and creamy dishes that are ubiquitous in many French restaurants. A wide variety of delicious salads and vegetable dishes should be on offer, alongside Puy lentil dishes and simply cooked meat and fish. Opt for these over anything creamy and avoid the bread basket. If you want dessert go for a simple fruit dish, such as a fruit salad – or ask for one to be prepared for you.

Mexican: This can be a tricky one, as many Mexican restaurants seem to serve tacos and cheese with everything. Obviously avoid dishes with lashings of sour cream and cheese, and also refried beans and wraps. However, Mexican restaurants should offer a variety of healthy bean and chickpea dishes, as well as grilled chicken and fish dishes. Black bean dishes are a good choice, as black beans are rich in antioxidants. Chilli non carne (bean rather than meat chilli) is also a good option – just ask that it isn't served with tacos and a cheese topping.

Seafood: Once every now and again is the rule with seafood. It's low in fat, but can be high in chemicals, and, of course, try to make sure it's as fresh as possible.

Boost your weight loss

When you've been following the life-changing weight loss plan for three or four weeks and you've dropped a few kilos, you may feel you want to boost your weight loss by doing a turbo weight-loss detox day.

The turbo weight-loss detox day is based on juice fasting. Fasting is an excellent way to remove unwanted toxins and weight very quickly and has been around for centuries. It is based on the principle that digestion takes up the vast majority of a body's energy, so when this energy is freed up it is used to heal, rejuvenate and rebalance the body. It's what your body does naturally when you're fighting off an illness, because by reducing your appetite it obtains more energy for dealing with the illness.

Juice fasting works best, because fresh juices provide the energy needed for optimum detoxification. Rather than starving the body, a juice fast feeds the system with high levels of vitamins and minerals, so during a juice fast, the body has a chance to eliminate even greater amounts of toxins.

By integrating this tool into your lifestyle you can avoid the usual side-effects of stress, such as weight gain, sleepless nights, fatigue, lowered immunity and feeling down. It's the ultimate pick-me-up and you may want to use it about once a month or more often if you're under heavy emotional or physical demands.

Don't go to work on a turbo weight-loss detox day. Pick a Saturday or Sunday, take a special day off work or clear your responsibilities for 24 hours to help your body rest and your mind gain as much as possible from the process. Use the timetable opposite as a guideline only. As long as you consume the correct amount of juice over the course of the day, you can take things at a pace that suits you. Read that book you've wanted to read for ages, relax with a massage or just enjoy peace of mind and body.

Turbo weight-loss detox day schedule

• Each juice meal should consist of one small glass of freshly made juice, made from fresh seasonal fruits of your choice (see page 151 for booster recipe suggestions).
• With each juice meal consume one teaspoon of psyllium husks, as this helps to reduce appetite and increase the elimination of toxic waste.
• Consume at least four litres of water and two mugs of vegetable broth (see page 151 for recipe) or miso soup in the course of the 24 hours.
• Drink as much herbal tea as you want.
• Don't do the turbo weight-loss detox for any longer than 24 hours, as longer term juice fasting requires management from professionals.

Time	Event
7.30	Cleansing drink of hot water and lemon
8.30	First juice meal
10.30	Herbal tea
12.00	Second juice meal
13.30	Vegetable broth or miso soup
15.00	Third juice meal
18.00	Fourth juice meal
19.00	Vegetable broth or miso soup
20.00	Fifth juice meal
20.30	Herbal tea
21.00	Epsom salts bath

If you really want to nutrient-max your diet to boost weight loss, but can't face the full turbo weight-loss detox, then spend at least a day trying to eat as many raw foods as you can. Keeping food in its natural state maintains the vitamin, mineral, amino acid and enzyme content, and foods such as vegetables, fruits, nuts, seeds, grains, sprouts, sprouted beans and fresh juices are all super-nutritious when consumed raw. The extra recipes at the back of the book will give you some ideas, but even the addition of a side salad and a few extra pieces of fresh fruit to your daily food routine can really make a difference.

The other thing you can do is eat lots of liver-loving foods, such as eggs and cruciferous vegetables like cabbage, for a couple of days. As your liver is your detoxifying and fat-metabolising organ, your body's detox and weight loss capabilities will receive a real helping hand. A good detox support formula can also have a dramatic effect (see Resources, page 157).

Wash away those cares

Detoxing needn't be hard work! Relaxing in a lovely warm bath of Epsom salts will help to draw out toxins from your blood and take the stress off your liver and kidneys. Epsom salts are magnesium sulphate, a naturally occurring mineral that has been used since the 17th century for purging and healing, and they can be bought at minimum cost from any chemist. Preparing a bath is easy – simply add 500g of Epsom salts to your bath water. Make sure the water is a comfortable temperature without being overly hot and don't use soap as it will interfere with the action of the salts. You can enhance the experience with candles and relaxing music. Try to keep warm and rest for at least one hour afterwards.

Caution: If you have high blood pressure or any heart condition you should not have an Epsom salts bath. If you have any joint pain, just use 100g of the salts.

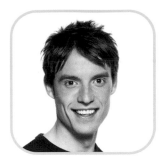

For the mind: Lifting your mood

Life moves through cycles. It's normal to have some days when you feel full of energy and optimistic, and other days when you feel more tired and pessimistic. If you notice you're having a 'down day' then instead of reaching for comfort food to bring you back up, I'd like to suggest a couple of healthier ways to lift your mood.

Your thoughts fuel your feelings, so you can use your thoughts to help you feel good by thinking about things that you are grateful for – I call this developing an attitude of gratitude! You can do this by simply reflecting on all the good things about your current body and life. Get into the habit of taking a couple minutes each day to write down ten things you're grateful for. Do your best to try to think of ten new things every day. This simple daily practice will train your brain to make you consciously aware of all the good things in your life, and you'll notice that your mood will naturally and effortlessly improve, day on day. You may also notice your overall health improving, because emotions of gratitude have been found to be very healing for the body.

You can also lift your mood in a matter of moments by changing your posture, facial expression, breathing and so on. You are wired to feel certain emotions when you do certain things with your body. If you notice yourself experiencing any negative emotions that could trigger comfort eating, whether it's boredom, sadness, loneliness or guilt, then make a positive physical change. Here are some suggestions for changing your body physiology to make yourself feel better.

Body part	Action
Eyes	Look up
Chin	Stick it up and out
Face	Put a big smile on it
Shoulders	Pull them back
Chest	Puff it up and out
Arms	Raise them above your head with palms facing the sky
Stomach	Breathe in deeply
Legs	Place them firmly a shoulders' width apart and stand tall

The 3Cs

Another effective way of getting rid of negative emotions and feeling more calm is to practise 3C vision by doing the following:

• Pick a spot on a wall to look at it, preferably above eye level, so that as you look at it, it feels as though your vision is bumping up against your eyebrows. Make sure your eyes are not so high that you cut off your field of vision.
• As you stare at the spot on the wall, let your mind go loose and focus all your attention on the spot. At this point you may find yourself wanting to breathe in and out deeply. Let yourself do so.
• Notice that within a matter of a few moments your vision will start to spread out, and you will begin to see more in the peripheral than in the central part of your vision. It will feel natural to take another couple of deep breaths in and out, so do that.
• Now, pay more attention to the peripheral part of your vision than to the central part of your vision. Notice colours, shadows, shapes and so on.

• Continue for as long as you want, while noticing how it feels. You will find calm, confident and content feelings come to you.

With a little practice you will be able to use 3C vision during your day-to-day life, whenever you want to feel calm, confident or content.

Harnessing the mind–body connection

Remember, your unconscious mind is linked with your autonomic nervous system, which is in charge of regulating many of your bodily functions. Your mind and body are also connected via your emotions. On top of that, your individual cells are designed to adapt themselves, based upon the messages sent to them by your brain. This all means that it is possible to change your body through the powerful combination of creating positive images in your mind and associating these images with positive feelings. I call the following exercise feelingisation.

• Relax: Start be ensuring you are not in fight or flight mode by taking a few moments to balance your breathing (see page 74).
• Feelingise: Now consider how you will know you've got the body and life you want. Imagine what you will see, hear, feel, smell and taste. Tune into the kinds of happy and celebratory thoughts you will be having. Do your best to associate strong positive feelings with the images in your mind.

I recommend you 'feelingise' for a few minutes every day to send consistent slimming messages from your brain to your body.

Enjoying more peace (even with a busy mind!)

If you want to take the mind–body connection further, I suggest you try meditation. When you still your mind, you still your body, allowing it to function more effectively. The remarkable thing about meditation is that by slowing down your mind you can actually speed up weight loss.

Meditation need not be difficult. Practised correctly it can be surprisingly simple.

• Be comfortable: many people like to sit cross-legged to meditate but it certainly isn't a prerequisite. You can do it very well in the comfort of your own home on a seat, sofa or even lying on your bed. Choose somewhere you won't be disturbed. Once you're perfectly comfortable, gently close your eyes and let your mind go loose. It may help to begin by imagining placing a warm smile on the top of your head and letting it melt down through your mind and body, soothing and softening your entire being as it melts all the way down and out of the bottoms of your feet.

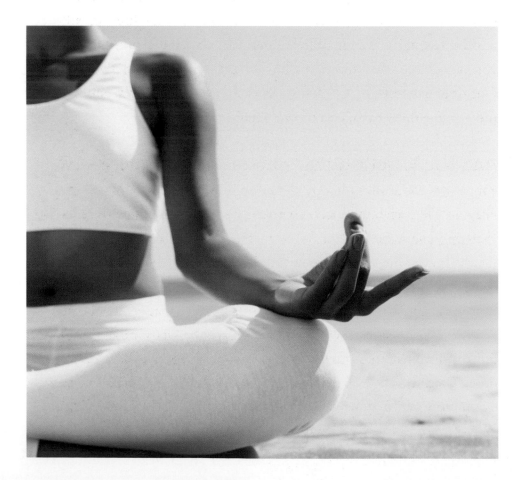

- Accept everything: Continue to meditate by observing your thoughts as if they are passing clouds in the sky. Never resist thoughts, as they are a natural by-product of your mind. By accepting them completely you lower the stress impact your thoughts have upon your body.
- Prioritise peace: It makes sense to think thoughts that have a positive impact on your mind and body, and you can enhance your meditative experience by occasionally thinking positive thoughts such as 'all is well' or 'I am loved.' It doesn't matter if you don't necessarily believe the positive thought yet, because it will still help your body to lose weight every time you prioritise peace by thinking peaceful thoughts.

Ideally, I recommend ten to 20 minutes of meditation two or three times every day – before you get out of bed in the morning, in the early evening and just before bed. Regular, short stints of meditation will make it easy for you to maintain a relaxed and positive mindset, reduce your stress levels and speed up your weight loss. However, if you can't find time to sit down and close your eyes, it will still help if you repeat the positive thoughts silently to yourself.

And finally, getting back on track if you ever fall off

You always do the best you can in the face of whole range of new and unexpected life circumstances. There will be times when the process of changing your habits and losing weight will be easy and enjoyable, and there may be times when you may revert back to your old ways. If you end up having what you consider a 'bad day' in respect to your eating, exercise or emotions, the most important thing you can do is be easy on yourself.

Use the bad day as an opportunity to remind yourself of your motives for losing weight, reconnect your end-goals with positive emotions by doing a feelingisation (see page 135), relax by setting the stress you're causing yourself free (see page 75) and rejoice by treating yourself to a healthy snack or meal that you really like. After all, one of the best gifts you can ever give yourself is to love yourself unconditionally.

More weight-loss plan recipes

Each of these recipes has been designed to be nutritionally balanced, easy to prepare but most of all tasty! The more variety and flavour in your diet, the easier it is to stick to healthy food. Enjoy!

Lunches

Spicy Lentil and Crème Fraîche Soup

SERVES 2

50g (1³/₄oz) red split lentils, rinsed

1 onion, chopped

1 carrot, chopped

600ml (1 pint) vegetable stock

1 bay leaf

¹/₂ tsp curry powder

¹/₄ tsp thyme

black pepper

1 tbsp crème fraîche

1. Place all the ingredients apart from the crème fraîche in a saucepan and bring to the boil. Simmer for 30 minutes.
2. Remove the bay leaf and blend the soup.
3. Stir in the crème fraîche and serve.

Split Pea and Chive Soup

SERVES 4

3 tbsp chives, chopped coarsely

3 tbsp natural yogurt

2 tbsp olive oil

1 onion, chopped

1 large carrot, peeled and chopped

2 garlic cloves , minced

255g (9oz) dried yellow or green split peas, picked over, rinsed
and drained

750ml (26fl oz) water

750ml (26fl oz) vegetable stock

1/4 tsp black pepper

a few chives

1. To make the chive cream, combine the chives and yogurt in a blender or
   food processor. Blend until smooth, cover and refrigerate until needed.
2. In a large saucepan, heat the olive oil over medium heat. Add the
   onion and sauté for about 6 minutes, until soft and lightly golden.
   Add the carrot and sauté for about 5 minutes, until soft. Add the garlic
   and sauté for 1 minute.
3. Stir in the split peas, water, stock and pepper and bring to a boil.
   Reduce the heat to low, cover partially and simmer for at least an
   hour, until the peas are tender.
4. In a blender or food processor, purée the soup in batches until smooth
   and return to the saucepan. Reheat gently.
5. Ladle into warmed individual bowls. Top each serving with a swirl of
   chive cream and a few long cuts of fresh chives. Serve immediately.

Chicken and Baby Potato Salad

SERVES 1

2 little gem lettuces, shredded

1 chicken breast, cooked with the skin on, cut into strips

3 small baby potatoes, boiled and chopped in halves

1 eating apple, cubed

5cm (2in) cucumber, sliced

6 baby plum tomatoes, halved

1 tbsp horseradish sauce or natural yoghurt

a few chives

1. Place the lettuce, chicken, potatoes, apple, cucumber and tomatoes in a bowl and mix together.
2. Dress with the horseradish sauce or yoghurt and chives.

Wholemeal Wrap with Mixed Peppers and Cottage Cheese

SERVES 2

1 tbsp olive oil

1 red pepper, deseeded and sliced thinly

1 green or orange pepper, deseeded and sliced thinly

1 yellow pepper, deseeded and sliced thinly

1 small red onion, sliced thinly

1 garlic clove, chopped finely

black pepper

4 tbsp cottage cheese

2 wholemeal wraps

1. Heat the olive oil in a wok-style pan, add the peppers, onion and garlic, and stir-fry gently for 6 minutes on a medium heat until the peppers are tender. Remove from heat and season with the black pepper.
2. Divide the cooked peppers and cottage cheese between the two wholemeal wraps, roll them up and serve.

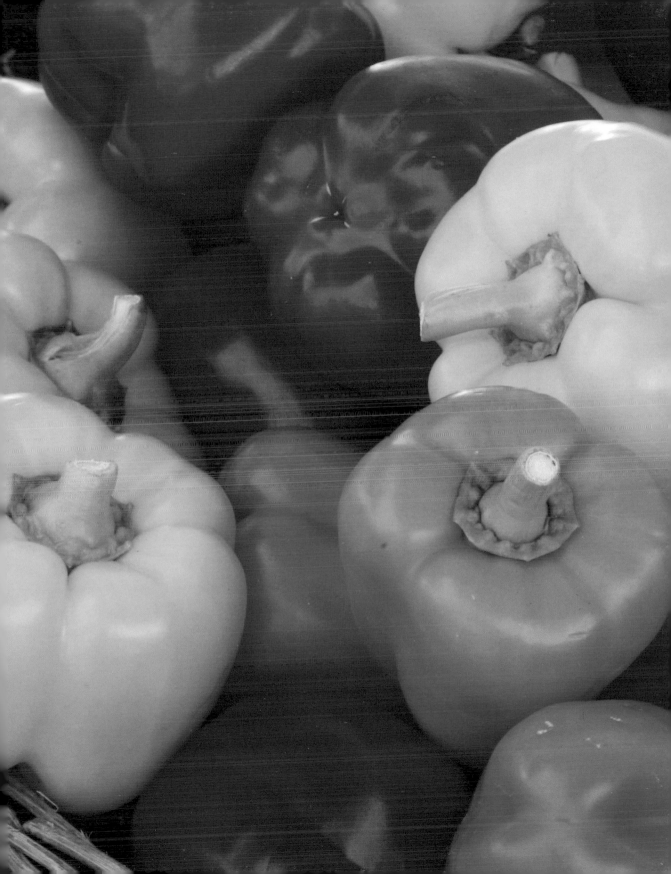

Avocado and Chicory Salad

SERVES 1

70g (2$^{1}/_{2}$oz) raisins or sultanas, or 5 fresh grapes, halved

$^{1}/_{2}$ celery stick, chopped

25g (1oz) walnuts, chopped

1 fresh chicory, chopped coarsely

$^{1}/_{2}$ avocado, peeled, pitted and diced

$^{1}/_{2}$ apple, cored and chopped or $^{1}/_{2}$ orange, peeled and chopped

1. In a large bowl toss together the raisins, sultanas or grapes, celery, walnuts and chicory leaves.
2. Fold in the avocado and fresh fruit.

Grilled Polenta and Goat's Cheese with Roasted Pine Nuts

SERVES 1

2 slices ready-to-cook polenta

200g (7oz) seasonal salad leaves

150g (5$^{1}/_{2}$oz) baby spinach leaves

1 carrot, grated

1 red onion, chopped finely

75g (3oz) sprouted mung beans

6 baby plum or cherry tomatoes, halved, or 4 sun-blush tomatoes, chopped

120g (4oz) goat's or sheep's cheese, cubed

1. Brush the polenta slices with oil and grill them for 5 minutes on each side.
2. Grill the goat's or sheep's cheese on a piece of baking parchment until lightly browned.
3. Combine all the remaining salad ingredients in a large bowl and place the polenta and goat's cheese on top.

Vietnamese Prawn Rice Paper Rolls

55g (2oz) raw prawns, chopped

1 handful of beansprouts

55g (2 oz) oyster mushrooms thinly sliced

1/2 bunch spring onions

1 handful of mint

1 handful of coriander

rice paper wrappers

6 tsp caster sugar

12 tbsp rice vinegar

3 tbsp sambal olek (spicy Indonesian sauce)

3 tbsp fish sauce

400ml (14fl oz) sunflower oil

2 handfuls of coriander

1. Very quickly blanch the prawns in boiling water to cook then refresh them in cold water.
2. In a large stainless steel bowl, gently mix together the beansprouts, oyster mushrooms, spring onions and fresh herbs.
3. Refresh the rice paper and then carefully sprinkle the filling into the centre of it, top with the prawn meat and roll carefully. The rolls can be stored for up to two hours on a tray lined with a damp cloth and covered with a damp cloth to prevent the rolls drying out.
4. To make the spring roll dipping sauce, mix the sugar and rice vinegar together until dissolved.
5. Fry the sambal for 2 to 3 minutes.
6. Place the sugar and rice vinegar, sambal, fish sauce, oil and coriander in a food processor and blend to a smooth sauce.
7. Pour the sauce into a saucer so that the rolls can be dipped in it.

Bottle and label the rest of the sauce, and keep it in a cool place.

Dinners

Smoked Haddock Kedgeree with Rocket and Sun-Blush Tomatoes

SERVES 1

150g (5^{1}/$_{2}$ oz) undyed smoked haddock fillet

100g (3^{1}/$_{4}$ oz) brown basmati rice

1 egg, hardboiled and chopped

3 sun-blush tomatoes, chopped

2 handfuls of rocket

black pepper

1 tbsp flaxseed oil

1. Place the fish in a pan with 75ml (2^{1}/$_{2}$ fl oz) of water, cover with a lid and steam for about 8 minutes.
2. Bring 250ml (8^{3}/$_{4}$ fl oz) of water to the boil and add the rice, cover with a lid and simmer for about 20 minutes or until light and fluffy.
3. Once the rice is cooked, fluff with a fork and stir in the fish, egg and sun-blush tomatoes. Either stir in the rocket or have it as a side salad.
4. Season with the black pepper and drizzle over the flaxseed oil.

Roasted Red Peppers with Goat's Cheese, Herbs and Pitta

SERVES 2

2 large red peppers, halved and seeded

2 courgettes, chopped

1 garlic clove, chopped

5cm (2in) chevre log goat's cheese

^{1}/$_{2}$ tsp thyme or rosemary

^{1}/$_{2}$ wholemeal pitta

2 handfuls of rocket

1 handful of olives

1. Preheat the oven to 200ºC/400ºF/gas mark 6.
2. Put the red pepper halves in an ovenproof dish, open side down, and cook for 30 minutes.
3. Lightly fry the courgette and garlic, removing from the heat before it's overdone.
4. Turn the red peppers over, spoon in the courgette mixture and bake for a further 10 minutes.
5. Top each pepper with a quarter of the chevre log, and sprinkle with the black pepper and thyme or rosemary.
6. Bake for 5 to 10 minutes, until the goat's cheese is lightly cooked.
7. Serve with the rocket, olives and toasted pitta.

Bun-Free Bean Burgers
SERVES 2

25g (1oz) sunflower seeds
340g (12oz) unsalted red kidney beans
1 small onion, chopped finely
1/2 tsp chilli powder
2 tbsp low salt ketchup
1 tbsp oatmeal or wheat germ

1. Preheat the oven to 180ºC/350ºF/gas mark 4.
2. Crush the sunflower seeds or chop them in a blender.
3. Mash the seeds and the beans together, and mix in the rest of the ingredients.
4. Transfer the mixture to an ovenproof dish and bake it for 20 minutes. Remove and allow it to cool.
5. Shape the mixture by hand into four smallish patties.
6. Return the patties to the oven and bake them for 15 minutes on each side.
7. Serve with a large green salad or steamed vegetables, and use a little extra tomato sauce on the side if you wish.

Cauliflower Curry

SERVES 2

1 tbsp olive oil

¹/₂ red onion, sliced

pinch of turmeric

pinch of cumin seeds

pinch of paprika

pinch of ground ginger

splash of white wine

2 tbsp tomato purée

splash of vegetable stock

2 tbsp red wine vinegar

2 tsp tomato ketchup

2 baby cauliflowers, chopped

1. Heat the oil in a pan and sauté the onion with all the spices for a few minutes.
2. Add the wine, tomato purée and stock, and heat for 3 to 4 minutes.
3. Stir in the vinegar, ketchup and cauliflower, and heat gently for 10 to 12 minutes.
4. Remove from the heat and serve at once.

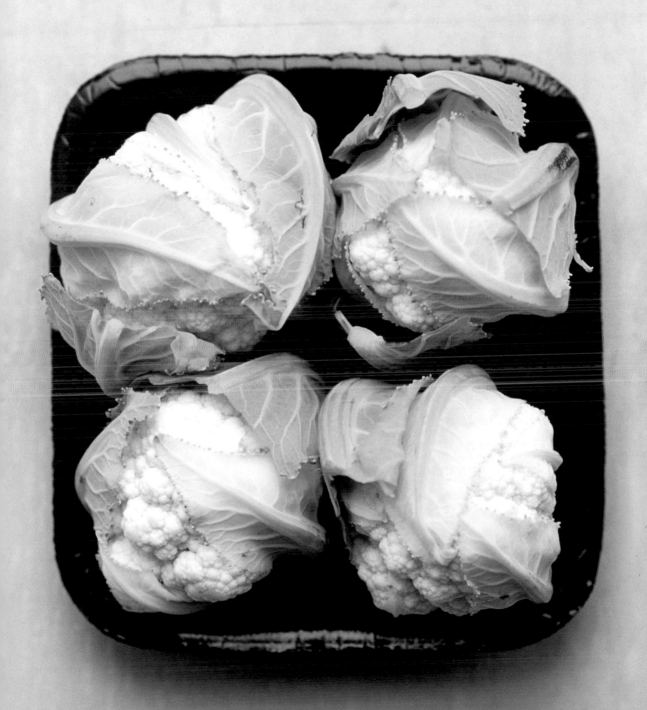

California Rolls

SERVES 2

2 sheets dried seaweed, cut in half

155g (5oz) sushi rice

1 tsp sesame seeds, toasted

1/4 cucumber, peeled, seeded and thinly sliced

1 tin salmon caviar

1 avocado, peeled, pitted and diced

1. Spread out the pieces of seaweed and divide the rice between them.
2. Sprinkle the toasted sesame seeds over the rice.
3. Place two slices of cucumber on each piece of seaweed, over the sesame seeds.
4. Divide the caviar into four and spread a portion over each set of cucumber slices.
5. Place the avocado over the caviar.
6. Using both hands, roll the seaweed up loosely, so the filling remains loose. Each roll should be about 10cm (4in) long.

Steamed Scallops with Chinese Shallots

SERVES 1

4 large scallops or 1 portion of white fish

2 tsp oyster sauce

2 baby red shallots, sliced finely

50g (1 3/4 oz) ginger, sliced finely

1 large red chilli, sliced finely

1/2 tbsp low sodium soya sauce

1 sprig coriander

1/2 teaspoon white pepper

1 tbsp sesame oil

1. Wash and clean the scallops, and smear them with the oyster sauce.
2. Stir-fry the shallots, ginger and chilli.
3. Steam the scallops until cooked and transfer them to a serving plate.
4. Cover the scallops with the cooked shallots, ginger and chillies, the soya sauce, coriander and a pinch of white pepper.
5. Heat the oil in a small, deep saucepan until almost smoking, then pour it over fish.

Avocado, Shiitake and Cashew Nut Spring Rolls

SERVES 2

$^1/_2$ avocado, peeled, pitted and diced

50g ($1^3/_4$ oz) shiitake mushrooms, chopped

1 small handful cashew nuts, chopped

50g ($1^3/_4$ oz) glass noodles, cooked and set aside

$^1/_2$ bunch spring onions, chopped

1 small handful of beansprouts

1 small handful of mangetout, cooked and set aside

$^1/_2$ red onion, chopped finely

1 tsp chilli sauce

$^1/_2$ tbsp flaxseed oil

4 spring roll wrappers

2 handfuls of mixed green leaves

1. Mix the avocado, mushrooms, cashew nuts, noodles, spring onions, beansprouts, mangetout and onion together.
2. Season with the chilli sauce and flaxseed oil.
3. Divide the mixture between the spring roll wrappers and roll up. Serve on the mixed leaves.

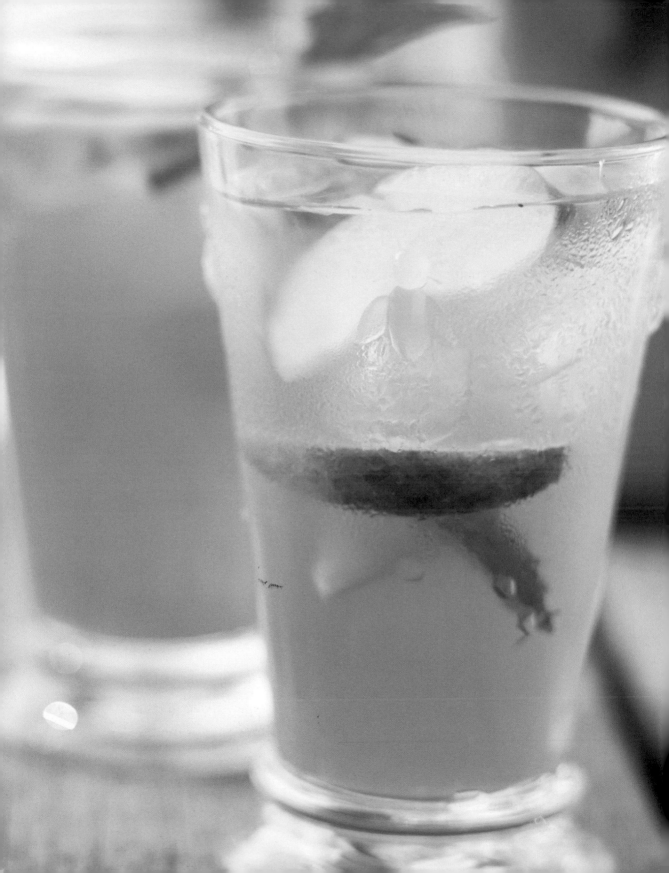

Juices, broth and raw recipes

Body Cleanser
SERVES 1
4 carrots, scrubbed
1/2 cucumber
1 apple, cored

Juice all the ingredients and drink at once.

Liver Lover
SERVES 1
2 carrots, scrubbed
1/2 beetroot

Juice all the ingredients and drink at once.

Digestive Cocktail
SERVES 1
1/4 lemon, unpeeled
1/2 grapefruit, peeled

Juice all the ingredients and drink at once.

Vegetable Broth
This broth is rich in minerals and vitamins. You can vary the taste by adding any spice except salt – cayenne pepper is especially good for a detox. The broth can be stored in the fridge for three days or frozen.

MAKES 2.8 LITRES (5 PINTS)
4 large potatoes, chopped
6 carrots, chopped

1 head of celery, including the leaves, chopped

1 handful of green vegetables, such as broccoli, kale or green beans, chopped

1 apple, cored and chopped

1 bunch fresh herbs, such as parsley, oregano or coriander, chopped

1. Put all the water, vegetables, apple and half the herbs into your largest pan. Bring to the boil then simmer gently for a minimum of 1^1/$_2$ hours or up to 3 hours for a more intense flavour.
2. Remove from the heat, strain off all the vegetables and fruit, and discard them.
3. Add the remaining herbs before serving.

Apple and Pear Porridge

If you don't have a juicer, use organic fruit juice and grate in a fresh apple when you're ready to eat the porridge.

SERVES 1

3 medium apples

2 pears

90g (3^1/$_2$ oz) rolled oats

40g (1^1/$_2$ oz) raisins

40g (1^1/$_2$ oz) almonds

^{1}/$_2$ tsp cinnamon

1. Cut the apples and pears into wedges and remove the cores. Juice the wedges to make about two small cups of juice. Keep the pulp.
2. In a medium-size bowl, combine the apple and pear juice and pulp with the oats, raisins, almonds and cinnamon. Mix well.
3. Cover the bowl and place in the refrigerator. Leave the raw porridge to soak overnight.

Superfoods Salad

This salad is easy to make and delicious to eat, but leave out the chilli if you prefer. It makes an excellent protein-packed lunch, which makes use of several superfoods.

SERVES 1

squeeze of fresh lemon juice

1/2 avocado, peeled, stoned and chopped

1 handful of sprouted beans, such as mung beans or alfalfa sprouts

1 handful of watercress or rocket leaves

1 tbsp flat-leaf parsley, chopped

5cm (2in) piece of cucumber, diced

3 spring onions, chopped finely

1/2 red pepper, deseeded and chopped finely

1 small red chilli, deseeded and chopped finely

1 tbsp apple cider vinegar

2 tbsp flaxseed oil or extra virgin olive oil

black pepper

1. Sprinkle the lemon juice over the avocado pieces and then put them, along with the beans, watercress, parsley, cucumber, spring onions, red pepper and chill into a bowl.
2. Put the vinegar, oil and black pepper into a screw-top jar and shake together vigorously. Pour over the salad and toss well.

Raw Veggie Casserole

SERVES 1

2 lettuce leaves

1 courgette

4 carrots

handful of cauliflower

handful of alfalfa sprouts

$1/2$ red pepper, deseeded and sliced

handful of chopped red cabbage

2 tomatoes

1 stalk of celery

2 carrots

juice of 1 lemon

1 handful of seeds or $1/2$ avocado

1. Place the lettuce leaves on a plate.
2. Shred the courgette, half the carrots, the cauliflower, sprouts, pepper and red cabbage in a food processor. Put them all in a large salad bowl and mix them together.
3. Blend the tomatoes, celery, other half of the carrots and lemon juice in a food processor. Then add the seeds or avocado and blend again until the mixture has the consistency of a moderately thick sauce.
4. Pour this sauce over the vegetables and serve on the lettuce.

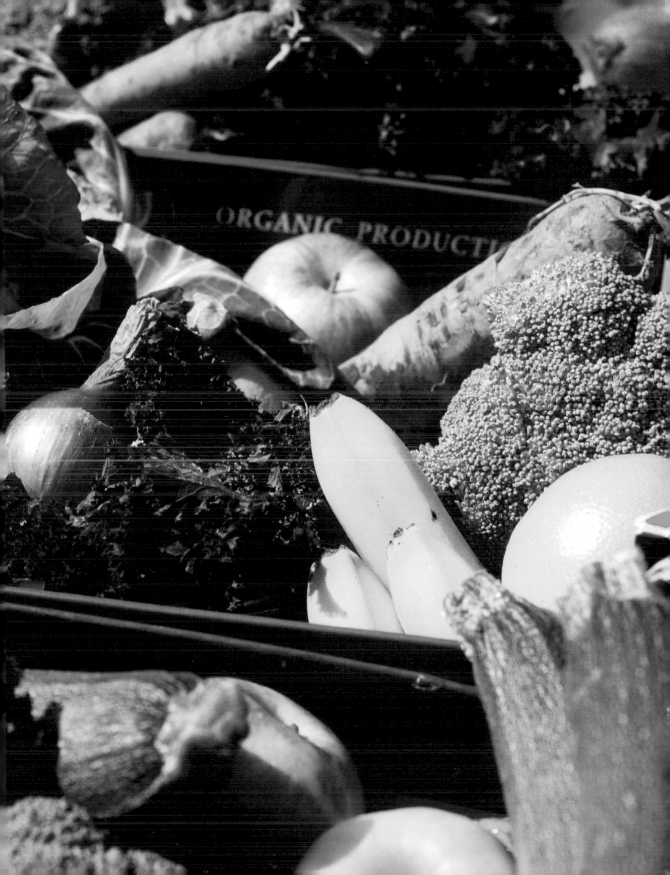

Resources

Amanda and Sandy

TV, books, events and online products relating to Amanda Hamilton:
www.amandahamilton.co.uk, tel: 0871 890 1331

Detox, weight loss and corporate health retreats with Amanda Hamilton
and her team: www.chrysalishealth.co.uk, tel: 0871 890 1331

Retreats, workshops, clinics and resources relating to Sandy Newbigging:
www.sandynewbigging.com, tel: 0131 208 4828

Mind Detox for health and happiness – events with Sandy Newbigging
and his team: www.minddetox.net, tel: 0131 208 4828

Products

Non-toxic household cleaning products from Mypure:
www.mypure.co.uk, tel: 0845 456 0639

Non-toxic household cleaning products from Ecover:
www.ecover.com

Alternatives to garden pesticides from Pesticide Action Network UK:
www.pan-uk.org, tel: 0870 241 6567

Natural skincare and cosmetics from Living Nature UK:
www.livingnature.com, tel: 01794 323 222

Natural skincare and body products from Napiers:
www.napiers.net, tel: 0131 343 3292

Food intolerance testing kits from Yorktest:
www.yorktest.com, tel: 0800 074 6185

Bragg liquid aminos, flaxseed oil and psyllium husks from
Your Health Store: www.yourhealthstore.co.uk

Flaxseed oil and flaxseed powder from the Flaxseed shop:
www.flaxseedshop.com, tel: 0871 233 2899

Yeast-free, gluten-free, low salt vegetable stock cubes from Goodness
Direct: www.goodnessdirect.co.uk, tel: 0871 871 6611

Amanda Hamilton's 7- and 14-day Home Detox Kits, and detox support formula (specialist liver supplement), from Nutrigold:
www.nutri-gold.com, tel: 0845 603 5675

Infrared sauna by Physiotherm from MagMed:
www.physiotherm.net, tel: 0845 225 5008

Juicers from Get Juicing: www.getjuicing.com, tel: 01952 277324

Organisations

British Association for Applied Nutrition and Nutritional Therapy:
www.bant.org.uk

Complementary Therapists Association:
www.complementary.assoc.org.uk, tel: 0870 201 1912

Federation of Independent Therapists: www.fit2practise.org

Books

Feinstein, D., Eden, D and Craig, G., *The Healing Power of EFT and Energy Psychology: Revolutionary Methods for Dramatic Personal Change*, Piatkus, 2006

Philips, A. and Philips, J., *The Powerwatch Handbook: Simple Ways to Make You and Your Family Safer*, Piatkus, 2006

Hamilton, A and Newbigging, S., *Life Detox: Clear Physical and Emotional Toxins from Your Body and Your Life*, Piatkus, 2007

Picture credits

Author photographs (pp10, 13, 18, 24, 45, 58, 69, 77, 83, 124, 133) by Adam Lawrence; p6 Richard Jung/Photolibrary; p9 Uli Pfeiffer/Photolibrary; p22 Bloom Image/Corbis; p33 Corbis/Photolibrary; p42 Tetra Images/Alamy; p50 Dex Image/Getty; P56 Tim Pannell/Corbis; p67 John Henley/Photolibrary; p85 Sam Stowell/Photolibrary; p89 Envision/Corbis; p93 James Baigrie/Photolibrary; p94, p101 Joy Skipper/Photolibrary; p107 Philip Wilkins/Photolibrary; p113 Matthew Doggett/Alamy; p117 Luzia Ellert/Getty; p118 James Baigrie/Photolibrary; p122 Ant Strack/Corbis; p136 Joaquin Palting/Corbis; p141 Aguilar Patrice/Alamy; p147 Bon Appetit/Alamy; p150 Debi Treloar/Redcover.com; p155 David Marsden/Photolibrary

Index

Note: page numbers in **bold** refer to illustrations, page number in *italics* refer to information contained in boxes and tables.